The Prostate

The Prostate

Facts and Misconceptions

by H. Salcedo, M.D., FACS

A Citadel Press Book
Published by Carol Publishing Group

Carol Publishing Group Edition, 1996

A Citadel Press Book
Published by Carol Publishing Group
Citadel Press is a registered trademark of Carol Communications, Inc.

Editorial Offices: 600 Madison Avenue, New York, NY 10022
Sales & Distribution Offices: 120 Enterprise Avenue, Secaucus, NJ 07094
In Canada: Canadian Manda Group, One Atlantic Avenue, Suite 105
Toronto, Ontario, M6K 3E7

Queries regarding rights and permissions should be addressed to:
Carol Publishing Group, 600 Madison Avenue, New York, NY 10022

Carol Publishing Group books are available at special discounts for bulk purchases, sales promotions, fund raising, or educational purposes. Special editions can also be created to specifications. For details contact: Special Sales Department, Carol Publishing Group, 120 Enterprise Ave., Secaucus, NJ 07094

Manufactured in the United States of America
10 9 8 7 6 5 4 3 2 1

Library of Congress Cataloging-in-Publication Data

Salcedo, H. (Hernando)
The prostate : facts and misconceptions / by H. Salcedo.
p. cm.
"A Citadel Press book."
ISBN 0-8065-1764-6
1. Prostate—Popular works. I. Title.
RC899.S25 1993 93-8840
616.6'5—dc20 CIP

Contents

Introduction

Diseases of the prostate constitute a major health problem for men. In fact, cancer of the prostate has become the most frequent cancer diagnosed in American men, and it ranks second behind lung cancer as the leading cancer killer in men. It is estimated that about 165,000 new cases of prostate cancer will be diagnosed this year (1993) in the United States, and although it is true that most men who have prostate cancer will die with the disease rather than from it, approximately 35,000 men will die from this dreadful disease in 1993 in the United States alone.

Diseases of the prostate, such as benign prostatic hypertrophy, cancer of the prostate, and prostatitis are very common in men. Yet many men know very little about the prostate gland—what it does, the problems related to it, and so on. There is a common misconception that prostate problems are limited to the aging man, yet many problems of the prostate occur in men between the ages of twenty and forty-five. Very few conditions in medicine cause more grief, anxiety, and fear, primarily because men feel it can lead to impotence, infertility, and even death.

This book was written in response to the great need to provide sound information about the prostate gland. It explains in detail the various diseases of the prostate, and provides information on symptoms of prostate diseases in order to encourage early diagnosis and cure. It also reviews the state-of-the-art technology being used today to diagnose and treat various diseases of the prostate, as well as current treatments under investigation.

It has not been until very recently that diseases of the prostate have been openly discussed. Thanks to the efforts of several public figures, celebrities, and U.S. senators who, themselves afflicted with prostate cancer, decided to go public and speak about their problem, the subject of prostate cancer has finally come out of the closet. Senator Robert Dole has recently appeared on nationally televised programs to speak about prostate cancer and to encourage early detection of the disease while it is still curable. This is the type of leadership needed to bring this killer disease to the attention of the public in the hope that with more awareness of its existence, more funds will be allocated for research, and more lives will be saved.

The Prostate

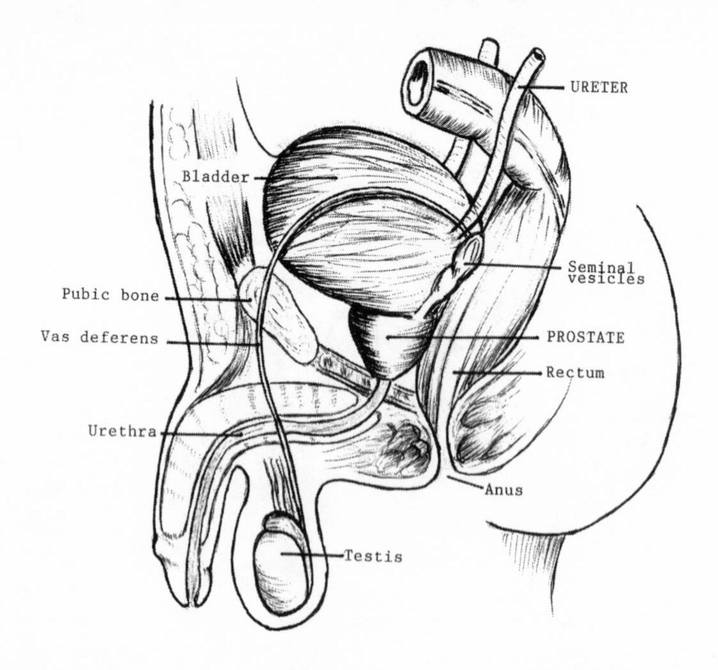

Figure 1-1. Lateral view of the prostate showing its relationship to the rectum, to the bladder, and to the urethra.

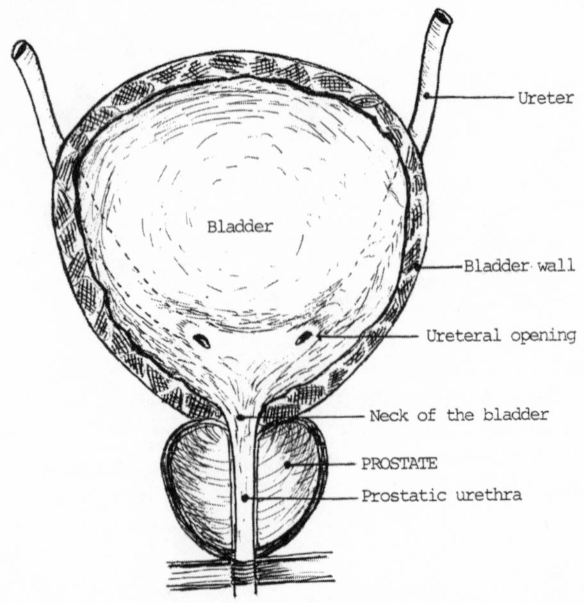

Figure 1-2. Anterior view of the prostate showing its relationship to the bladder and showing the urethra as it goes through the prostate.

CHAPTER 1

The Prostate

In order to be able to understand any problems that one might have with the prostate gland, some very basic knowledge of its anatomy and function will be helpful. The prostate gland in the adult male is roughly the size and shape of a chestnut and weighs about 20 grams, or a little less than one ounce. This relatively small gland, capable of causing so much grief, is situated in front of the rectum and just below the bladder, fitting like a collar around the **urethra** (Figs. 1-1, 1-2). The urethra is a long, muscular tube that carries urine from the bladder to the outside. It first passes through the prostate and then through the penis and ends at its opening, known as the **urethral meatus**. The part of the urethra that goes through the prostate is called the **prostatic urethra**, which may be obstructed as the prostate gland becomes enlarged with advancing age. The prostate is often likened to an apple with the core removed. The space left inside the apple after removal of its core would correspond to the prostatic urethra.

The prostate is not actually a single gland, but is composed of numerous tiny glands arranged in lobes that discharge their secretions into the urethra upon ejaculation. It is also composed of smooth muscle, blood vessels, and connective elastic tissue. It is surrounded by a dense and fibrous shell called the **capsule**.

The Male Urinary and Reproductive Systems

The urinary and reproductive systems are intimately connected and function in perfect synchronization. In order to appreciate the function of one system, it is important to understand the function of the other

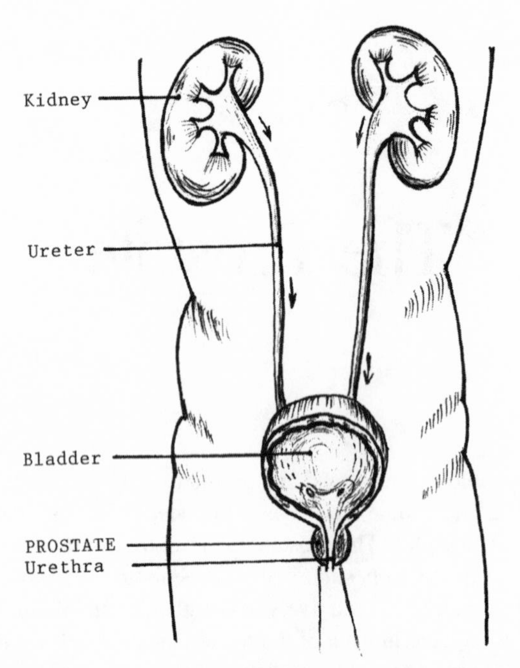

Figure 1-3. Urinary tract. The arrows show the direction in which the urine flows.

system as well. When problems develop in one of the systems, it will affect the other.

Urinary System

The kidneys are the organs responsible for filtering various waste products out of the blood; the result of this filtration is the production of urine, which contains chemical substances that would be toxic if they remained in the body. The urine produced by the kidneys travels down into the bladder through two long, narrow tubes called **ureters** (Fig. 1-3). The bladder is a powerful hollowed muscle that stores the urine which has been produced by the kidneys. It has three openings: two small ones that correspond to the ureters, and a larger one (or exit valve into the urethra) known as the neck of the bladder, or **vesical neck**. The neck of the bladder functions as the **internal sphincter**, or **bladder neck sphincter** (Fig. 1-4).

In men, there are actually two circular muscles, or sphincters: the one

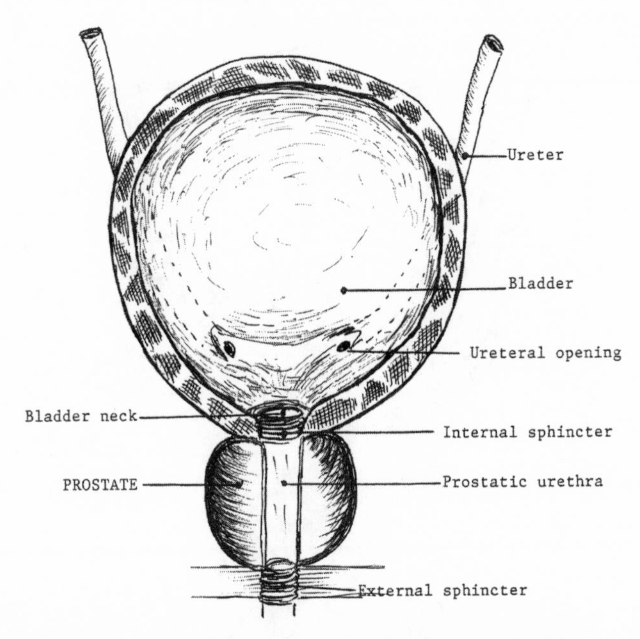

Figure 1-4. Anterior view of the prostate showing the internal sphincter, which wraps around the neck of the bladder, the external sphincter, and their relationship to the prostatic urethra, which goes through the entire prostate.

mentioned above and the other known as the **external sphincter**, which is located just below the prostate. The latter is the muscle you voluntarily contract when you want to suddenly stop the flow of urine while voiding. These two muscles are responsible for preventing urine leakage and work in perfect synchronization. At the moment of orgasm, the sphincter at the neck of the bladder closes and the lower sphincter relaxes. The semen, which enters the urethra under pressure, cannot enter the bladder and is thus forced down the urethra to the outside. The closure of the vesical neck also prevents urine from mixing with the semen.

Reproductive System

The reproductive system has various components, including the testes, which are located in the scrotum and have two principal functions. The testes manufacture the sperm cells, or **spermatozoa**, needed for procreation, and also produce the male hormone **testosterone**, which is

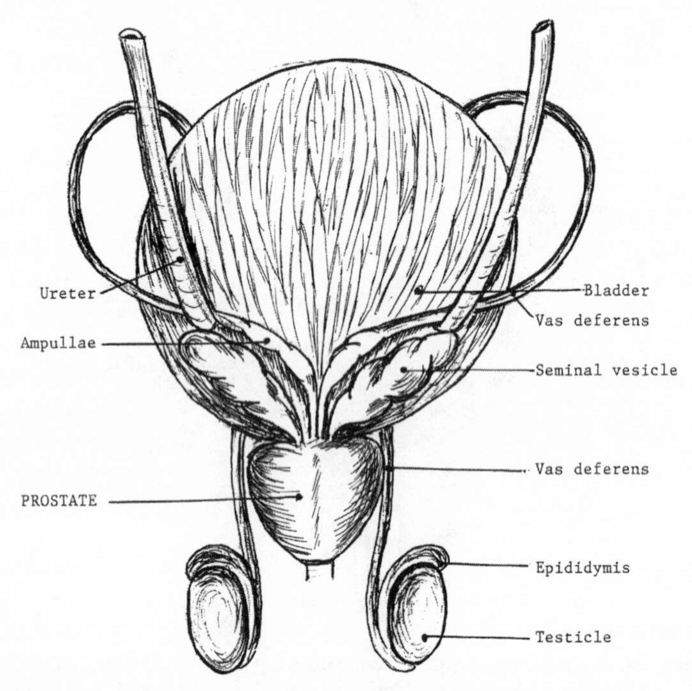

Figure 1-5. Posterior view of the prostate showing its relationship to the seminal vesicles, to the ampullae, and to the bladder. It shows also the testicles and the vas deferens.

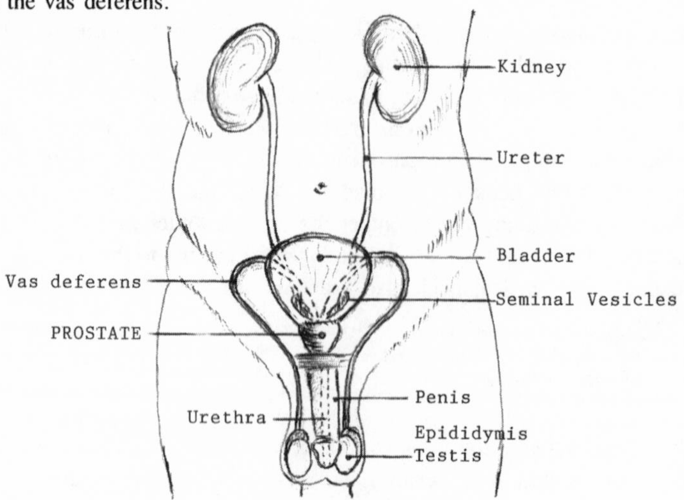

Figure 1-6. Frontal view of genital and urinary systems.

responsible for male sexual characteristics, such as the growth of a beard, changes in the pitch of voice, appearance of hair on the chest, baldness, etc.

The sperm cells produced by the testicles take about ten weeks to mature. They then leave the testes and enter the **epididymis** (a tubular structure attached to the testis), where they are stored for about three weeks. After the sperm has matured, it travels through the **vas deferens**, a long, narrow, heavily muscled tube attached to the epididymis (Fig. 1-5 and Fig. 1-6). Each vas deferens ends at a point called the **ampulla**. The sperm is stored in the ampullae until released during ejaculation. Next to the ampullae are the **seminal vesicles**; these are two small sacs about two inches long and half an inch wide, located just behind the bladder and in front of the rectum. They secrete a fluid containing fructose that is part of the semen and that is important for the survival of sperm cells.

During sexual stimulation, the penis becomes erect due to an increased flow of blood into the spongy tissues inside the penis. At the peak of sexual excitement orgasm takes place and strong muscular contractions propel spermatozoa and fluid from the prostate and each vas deferens into the prostatic urethra. The strong muscles that surround the base of the penis and urethra contract and force the semen to the outside, producing ejaculation, and at the same time the sphincter at the neck of the bladder closes and thereby prevents the fluid from entering the bladder.

What the Prostate Does

In spite of its importance, the prostate remains one of the most poorly understood glands in the human body. We know, however, that it has a sexual function but is only indirectly involved in procreation. The main function of the prostate gland is the production of part of the fluid that makes up the vast majority of the semen. The purpose of this prostate fluid is to serve as a vehicle to carry the sperm cells to the outside at the time of ejaculation. The prostate fluid contains a variety of enzymes, zinc, citric acid, fructose, substances that neutralize bacteria, and other substances important for protection of sperm cells. Thus, the prostate plays a significant role in the normal delivery of sperm during sexual intercourse.

A group of fluids produced by the prostate, called **prostaglandins**, have recently received significant attention as remarkable agents that

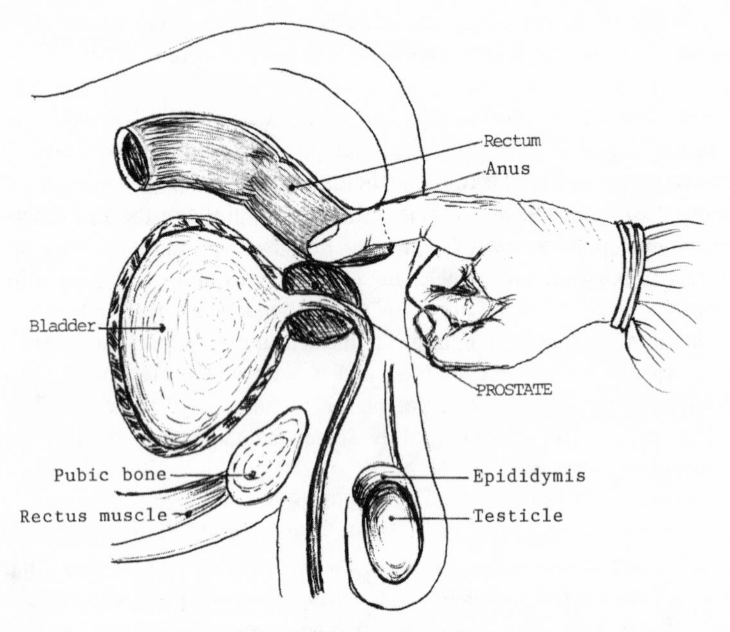

Figure 1-7. Digital rectal examination.

have effects on smooth muscle fibers and blood vessel walls. These have been used experimentally to produce dilatation of the neck of the womb and uterine contractions during childbirth. One of many theories about prostaglandins produced by the prostate is that they encourage the **cervix** (opening of the uterus) to dilate in order to facilitate the passage of the sperm through the cervix into the uterus so as to fertilize the egg. It would, therefore, seem logical that abnormalities of the prostate and seminal vesicle secretions could result in some cases of infertility. However, to date, the effects of seminal plasma on male infertility have not been well documented.

Age Changes in the Prostate

In the newborn, the prostate is a tiny organ, the size of a pea. It gradually increases in size until puberty, at which time changes occur very rapidly over a period of six to twelve months. During that period of time, it grows to more than twice its size. These changes are thought to be due to the secretion of the male hormone testosterone by the testes.

The growth of the prostate slows down until a man reaches his early thirties. In some men, after the age of forty-five or fifty, the prostate begins to grow again and slowly becomes enlarged, a process called **benign prostate hypertrophy**, or **hyperplasia (BPH)**. BPH is a process of aging during which the prostate enlarges, and it is often accompanied by various degrees of difficulty in voiding. Not all men have this growth and enlargement but many of them do, and not all men with enlargement develop symptoms of obstructed voiding, but many do. Why this is true is not well understood, but it appears to be an inherited trait.

How the Prostate Is Examined

Digital Rectal Examination (DRE)

The prostate is not easily accessible, and unfortunately a man cannot perform a self-examination, as women, who are advised to examine their breasts on a regular basis, are able to. **Digital rectal examination** is an examination performed by a physician. Since the prostate sits in front of the rectum, it lends itself to examination through the rectum. Wearing a rubber or plastic glove, the physician places the well-lubricated forefinger on the anal orifice and gently presses until the sphincter muscle of the anus relaxes. The finger is slowly inserted into the rectum, with the pad of the forefinger facing forward (Fig. 1-7). The examiner will feel the gland as an elastic bulging surface. Prostate consistency may be soft, hard, or fluctuant, and the size may be normal or enlarged. The doctor can also check for shape, symmetry, and for the presence of lumps or nodules. The prostate fluid that may drain into the urethra during the examination can be examined under the microscope for possible infection. The secret to avoiding discomfort during the examination is for the patient to relax the anal sphincter as much as possible, and the physician to be gentle with the examining finger.

It is widely recognized that the routine use of rectal examination is helpful in the early detection of cancer of the prostate, and that it represents the single most important phase of the physical examination for detecting this cancer.

CHAPTER 2

Benign Prostate Hyperplasia (BPH)

The "Gift" of Maturity

Benign enlargement of the prostate, known in medical terminology as benign prostate hyperplasia (or hypertrophy) and commonly referred to as BPH, is growth of the prostate that afflicts two species only: man and dog. The term "benign" means that it is not malignant; therefore, this condition neither spreads into nor attacks other organs, as cancer does.

Enlargement of the prostate occurs in most men over the age of forty-five or fifty. It is estimated by most researchers that this condition occurs in more than 50 percent of men over the age of fifty, in about 75 percent of those over the age of eighty, and in more than 90 percent of those over the age of ninety. Development of prostate enlargement (BPH) is, therefore, an almost universal feature of the aging man. As the prostate becomes enlarged, it protrudes into the base of the bladder, narrowing the urethra and causing obstruction to the flow of urine.

In order to understand clearly how BPH causes obstruction of the prostatic urethra, it may be helpful to liken the prostate to an apple with its core removed, as we did in Chapter 1. The space left inside the apple after removal of its core would correspond to the prostatic urethra. When BPH develops, the new growth of the prostate begins just below the lining of the prostatic urethra (Fig. 2-1). As this new growth slowly continues, usually over a period of years, it tends to grow in an outward as well as an inward direction (Fig. 2-2). When the growth occurs

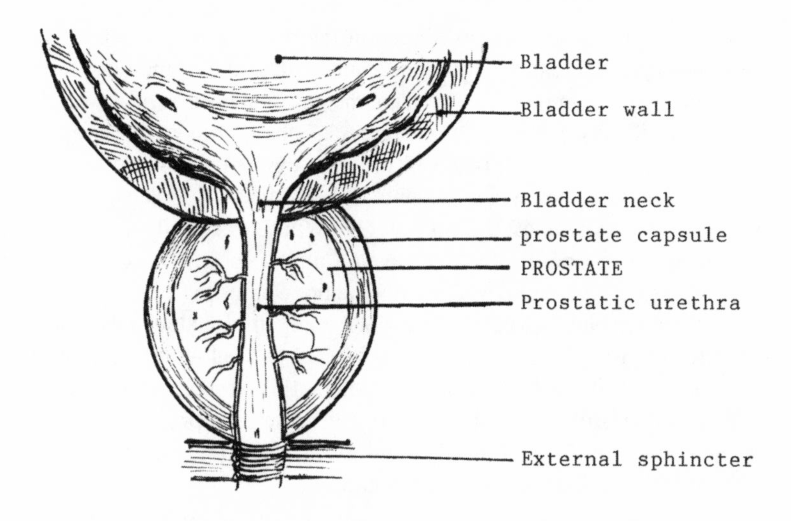

Figure 2-1. Above: Normal unobstructed prostate. Below: Early BPH. Note that the new growth of the prostate begins just below the lining of the prostatic urethra.

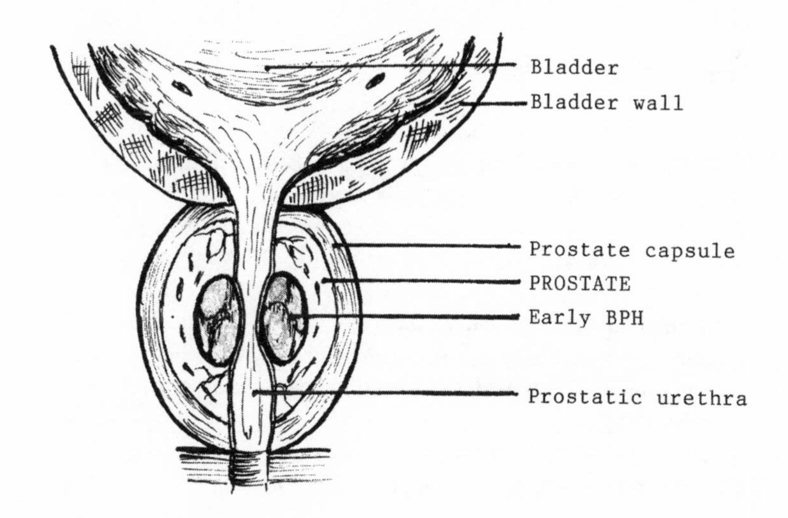

primarily only in an outward direction the prostate may reach a huge size and yet not cause any significant obstructive symptoms if the urethra is not compromised. When the growth occurs in an inward direction, it may cause varying degrees of obstruction of the prostatic urethra (Fig. 2-2), and it is this obstruction that is responsible for most of the symptoms for which patients consult their physicians.

The new growth of the prostate does not necessarily occur in a symmetrical manner. Sometimes even a moderate growth of the prostate gland may cause significant obstruction, as in the case of the so-called median lobe hypertrophy, where only the median lobe shows significant growth. Since this lobe is located just below the neck of the bladder, it will tend to protrude through this vesical neck, causing significant obstruction (Fig. 2-3). In this case, the prostate may feel normal in size on digital rectal examination, since this median prostate lobe cannot be felt on rectal examination.

The precise cause of BPH is not known and has been a source of speculation and great controversy for centuries. It is known that male hormones have a significant role in the development of BPH, but exactly how this happens is not clear.

Attempts to identify risk factors in men who develop BPH have not been successful. No relationship between this condition and factors such as celibacy, excessive sexual activity, stress, sedentary lifestyle, or other conditions has been established.

Symptoms of Obstructive BPH

BPH does not always cause symptoms. A good estimate is that about one-quarter to one-half of men who have BPH will also have enough symptoms to make them visit their physician.

Symptoms of obstructive BPH are grouped together under the term **prostatism**. These symptoms are generally:

- Urinary frequency and urgency
- Hesitancy or difficulty in starting the flow of urine
- Getting up from bed to urinate several times during the night (**nocturia**)
- Small caliber of the urinary stream
- Difficulty voiding, sometimes having to strain

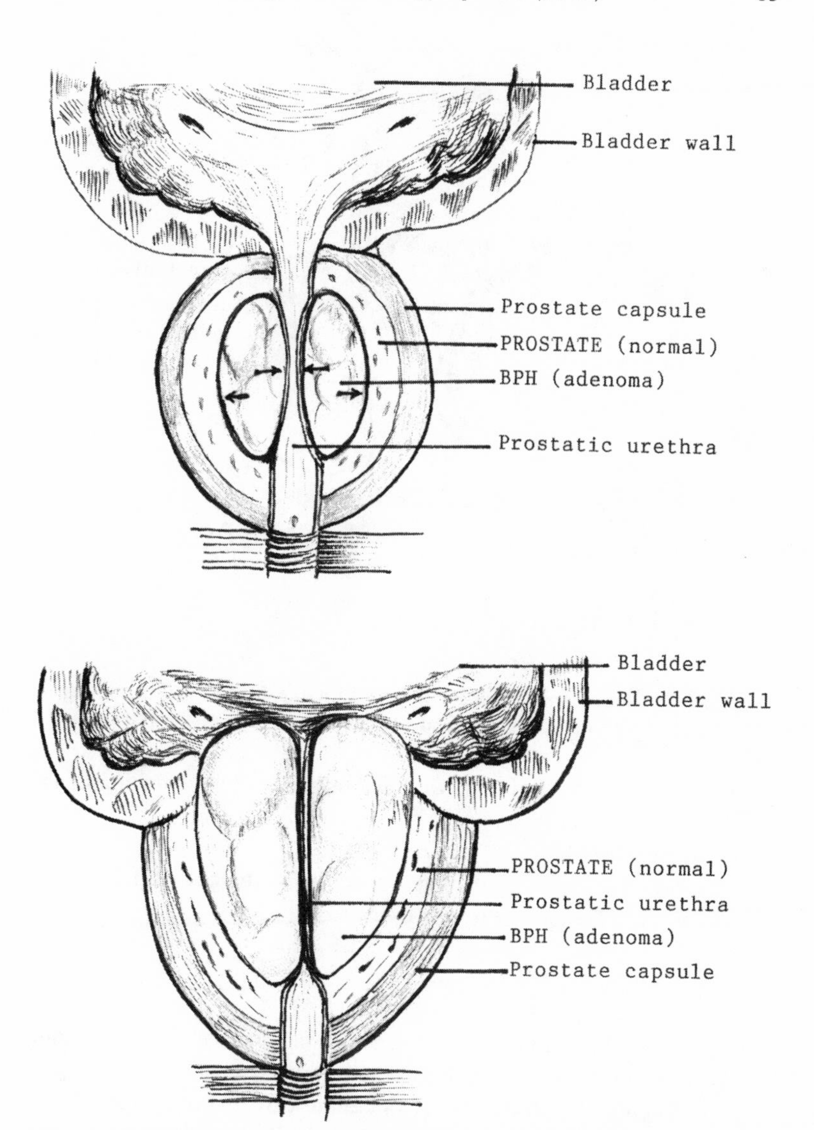

Figure 2-2. Further stages of BPH. Note how the urethra becomes progressively more obstructed by the expanding new prostate growth. The normal prostate tissue is compressed against the prostate capsule.

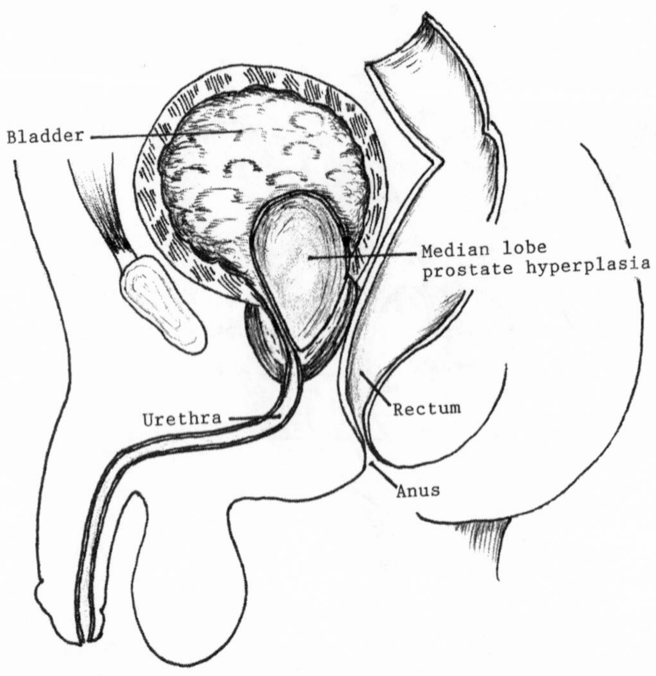

Figure 2-3. Severe obstruction of the neck of the bladder and the prostatic urethra by a significant enlargement of the median lobe of the prostate.

- Lack of satisfaction with voiding and incomplete emptying of the bladder
- Urinary dribbling
- Occasional presence of blood in the urine (**hematuria**)
- Urinary retention, in severe cases

Urinary Frequency

Frequency of urination depends on many factors: the amount of fluid intake, loss of body fluids due to perspiration, temperature, and ingestion of diuretics, such as drinks containing caffeine or alcohol. These diuretics make the kidneys produce increased amounts of urine, and normally a person will have to urinate more often after ingesting them.

Men with obstructive BPH often have to urinate frequently, because they are unable to empty their bladder completely and the bladder reaches its capacity more quickly. An obstructed bladder can develop irritability and signals fullness at smaller volumes. Patients who have obstructive BPH are instructed by their physicians to avoid ingesting caffeine or alcohol, because their urinary frequency becomes more severe. Urinary frequency is often associated with **urgency**, which is the acute desire to urinate, sometimes accompanied by a sensation of impending leakage.

Hesitancy

Hesitancy is the term used to indicate an abnormal delay between the initiation of the voiding act and the beginning of the flow of urine. Eventually the flow of urine starts, but the stream is usually weak and without force. In normal individuals, this time lapse is only a few seconds. However, in public places this may be longer, as psychological inhibition may occur. Patients with prostate obstruction tend to have hesitancy, which may vary from a few seconds to several minutes. The cause of hesitancy is not clear, but it appears to be due to the time needed to attain the necessary pressure within the bladder to overcome the increased resistance caused by the obstruction.

Small Caliber of the Urinary Stream

Obstructive changes usually occur gradually, and some patients may not be aware of the small caliber of the urinary stream. They may notice sometimes, that compared with other males, the voiding process takes longer. Voiding flow rates measure the caliber of the urinary stream and are very useful in the evaluation of treatments for BPH.

Nocturia

Being awakened during sleep by the desire to urinate is known as nocturia. Most normal men will occasionally experience nocturia if they drink large volumes of liquid before they go to sleep, or if they drink alcohol or coffee late at night. The number of times that men with obstructive BPH are awakened with the desire to urinate varies with the degree of obstruction. In severe cases, however, this may occur as often as every hour or less. Nocturia is thought to be related to the obstruction, and incomplete emptying which produces irritability of the bladder.

Lack of Satisfaction With Voiding

A feeling of incomplete emptying is a common urinary symptom. It is generally felt as mild pressure or discomfort in the lower part of the abdomen (bladder area) or may be a feeling of further desire to void after voiding has ended. Normal individuals void and empty the bladder completely, but when obstruction develops, only a limited amount of urine is evacuated with each voiding, so that when the person has finished and thinks his bladder is empty, a certain amount of urine remains there. The amount of urine left in the bladder after voiding has ended is known as **residual urine**. It is important to determine the amount of residual urine, because it helps the physician evaluate the degree of obstruction present. Difficulty voiding is a very common symptom of obstructive BPH, and is closely related to the small caliber of the urinary stream. The obstructed male feels urines does not flow easily and he frequently finds himself having to strain to increase the force of the stream.

Urinary Dribbling

Normally, at the end of voiding, the urinary flow ends abruptly. In the obstructed male, the flow may continue at a lower pressure for a few more seconds. This seems to occur because the bladder pressure falls toward the end of urination, and the increased resistance offered by the enlarged prostate will prevent a continuous flow. Sometimes, the bladder contracts again (in an effort to empty completely) after the patient thinks he has finished voiding, thus causing dampening of his underwear. This is both a cause of worry and an embarrassment for most males with prostate obstruction. From time to time a certain amount of dribbling may occur at the end of urination. This is due to a small amount of urine that is retained in the urethra, after the bladder neck closes. Patients with dribbling are generally advised to wait a few seconds longer at the end of urination to allow the remaining drops of retained urine to drain.

Hematuria

The term hematuria means that blood is present in the urine. An enlarged prostate sometimes has dilated small surface veins that may break and bleed. Hematuria should always be investigated because of the possibility of associated bladder tumor or other serious conditions of the urinary tract.

Urinary Retention

Acute urinary retention is the inability to pass water at all. It is an alarming condition that causes significant distress and pain and requires prompt medical attention. Drinking alcohol sometimes triggers an attack of acute retention. Certain drugs, such as decongestants (used against common colds) and antihistamines (used against allergies), may cause a similar effect. Acute urinary retention may also occur in the older male after surgical procedures. The medications given prior to administration of anesthesia to dry up secretions (known as anticholinergics) tend to relax the bladder and interfere with its proper functioning. Another cause of retention after surgery may be the administration of painkillers. These drugs dull the normal sensation of bladder fullness, and if the bladder becomes overly distended, it is unable to contract effectively and empty well. Urinary retention does not always occur suddenly. It may develop gradually over a period of months or even years. The patient voids frequently in very small amounts and may not even be aware that there is a problem. As his bladder gradually becomes more and more distended, he may notice some swelling of the lower part of the abdomen that he may attribute to lack of activity or overweight.

The author has had the opportunity to see many such cases; the instances are not infrequent and are sometimes discovered accidentally during an X-ray examination. Occasionally, a patient has gone to surgery for exploration of an abdominal mass that, to the surgeon's embarrassment, turned out to be nothing more than a full bladder. These days cases of "silent retention" are not likely to occur, thanks to the availability of modern tests, such as abdominal sonograms and CT scans, and other diagnostic tools that are now used routinely.

Effects of BPH

Effects of BPH on the Bladder

In the act of voiding, the contraction of the entire bladder forces urine down the urethra to the outside. Whenever there is an obstruction, such as one caused by BPH, the bladder muscle has to work much harder in

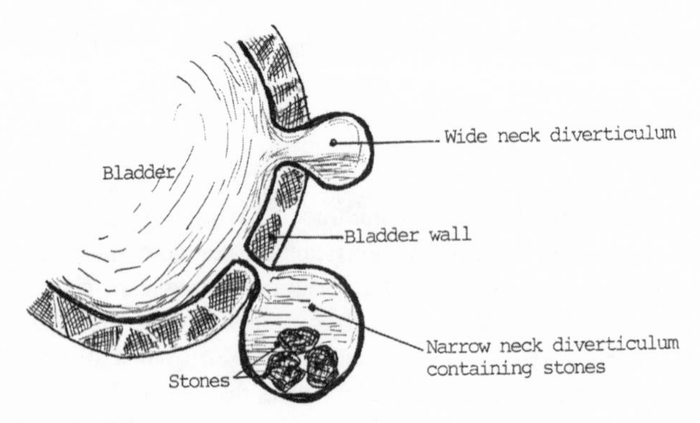

Figure 2-4. Different types of diverticula. These diverticula are the result of chronic bladder outlet obstruction.

order to do its job of emptying itself during voiding. When the bladder has to work harder and contract more forcefully to overcome the increased resistance caused by the obstruction, the bladder muscle undergoes thickening of its wall, in much the same manner that any muscle enlarges when it works harder. As the obstruction process continues, the bladder becomes very thick and irregular in its inner surface. This appearance of the interior of the bladder is known as **trabeculation**, and is characterized by the presence of irregular crossing bands of enlarged muscle. The thickening of these muscle bands leaves areas of weakness, through which the lining of the bladder may herniate the form pouches, which can be likened to the beginning of a blowout in a tire tube (Fig. 2-4). These pouches or pockets, known as **diverticula**, generally do not cause problems if they are small or if they have wide necks, but the large ones with narrow necks may not drain properly and may cause stones to form, which can lead to chronic infection and bleeding and may need to be removed surgically.

Prolonged stasis of urine in the bladder may cause stones to form. Bladder stones cause irritation and trauma to the bladder interior and sometimes cause further obstruction, as they tend to gravitate toward the neck of the bladder during voiding. Occasionally a small stone may actually pass through the vesical neck and get stuck in the urethra, causing very acute symptoms.

Bladder stones vary in size from a few millimeters in diameter to the size of an orange. Very large stones generally require removal through an incision in the bladder, while small ones may be removed through the urethra.

Effects of BPH on the Ureters

The ureters are the channels that carry the urine from the kidneys into the bladder. Most cases of uncomplicated bladder outlet obstruction presented to the urologist do not show any significant change in the ureters or kidneys. In some cases, however, when the bladder does not empty properly and becomes distended, the pressure in the ureters becomes higher, the ureters don't empty well, and they dilate. The wall of the ureters becomes overstretched, loses muscle tone, and becomes unable to contract rhythmically to propel urine into the bladder (Fig. 2-5).

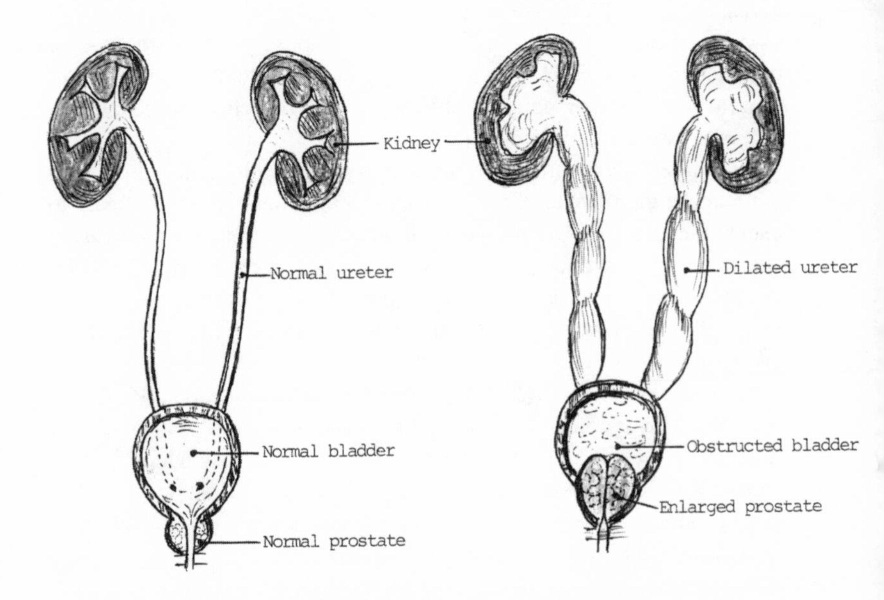

Figure 2-5. Normal urinary tract (left) compared to a badly obstructed urinary tract as a result of prostate enlargement (right). In cases of obstruction of the bladder by BPH, the kidneys and ureters cannot drain properly and the increased pressure makes them become dilated.

Effects of BPH on the Kidneys

As the obstruction of the bladder continues and the ureters become dilated, the kidneys cannot empty properly. If high pressure builds up in the ureters, the kidneys dilate and can no longer filter out the harmful toxins efficiently. As a result, kidney failure develops, causing uremic poisoning, or uremia (a serious condition that is fatal if not treated promptly).

How Obstructive BPH Is Diagnosed

Clinical History and Physical Examination

The most important step in diagnosing obstructive BPH is obtaining a good clinical history. The patient is asked about his symptoms and is given an opportunity to discuss in detail all of his complaints. This alone will allow the physician do draw a bead on the presence of obstruction due to BPH. The physician will take note of any previous or present illnesses or medical problems such as diabetes, cardiovascular diseases, urinary problems, etc.

Digital rectal examination is the only part of the physical examination that checks the prostate directly. This examination is done routinely to check the prostate for presence of nodules or areas of **induration** (firmness), but it does not help in the diagnosis of obstructive BPH. Digital rectal examination can check only the back of the prostate, and although it gives the physician a rough idea of the size of the prostate, it cannot determine the exact size.

Examination of the abdomen is done by having the patient lie flat on his back. The abdomen is examined for masses, areas of tenderness, or fullness of the bladder. It is not unusual to find a distended bladder, which is at times palpable up to the navel, in cases of a retention. The genitals are also checked for structural abnormalities, gross alterations from "normal," and tenderness.

Blood Tests

No known blood test diagnoses BPH, but there are blood tests that are commonly used to measure kidney function. The usual test measures **creatinine**, a substance eliminated by the kidneys. When the kidneys function normally, the blood creatinine level is normal. Abnormal elevation of creatinine generally indicates a decrease in kidney function, but this is not necessarily permanent. The blood creatinine level may be elevated because the kidneys cannot function normally in the face of obstruction. Once the obstruction is removed the urine flows normally again, the blood creatinine level frequently returns to normal, oftentimes within a few days. Normal creatinine levels vary somewhat with age and muscular development, but in the adult, the levels are generally between 0.5 and 1.5 ml/per 100 cc of blood.

Urine Tests

Examination of the urine is a very simple study that gives the physician a great deal of information. Although a urine analysis does not diagnose BPH, it will help in the diagnosis of other conditions of the urinary tract that may be occurring at the same time. It may detect the presence of sugar in a diabetic patient. The presence of large amounts of protein in the urine may suggest significant kidney disease. When blood is present in the urine, further investigation is necessary, as this may be indicative of the presence of a malignant tumor or other serious condition of the urinary system. A urine analysis may also suggest the presence of infection, which may be confirmed by taking what is known as a "culture" of the urine. A sample of urine is placed on a small dish containing nutrients on which bacteria will grow. This dish is placed in an incubator at a temperature suitable for bacterial growth. After twenty-four hours of incubation bacteria present in the urine can be identified and the number of bacterial colonies can be counted. At the same time, the bacteria are exposed to small disks impregnated with different antibiotics to see which of them are the most effective against the bacteria that may be growing.

There are other tests that will help the physician to arrive at the diagnosis of obstructive BPH, such as:

Excretory Urogram

Also known as intravenous pyelogram or simply as IVP, this is an X-ray study that provides the physician with a great amount of information about the entire urinary tract. Since an X ray of the abdomen shows only the bones and some of the soft tissues, a liquid substance is injected into

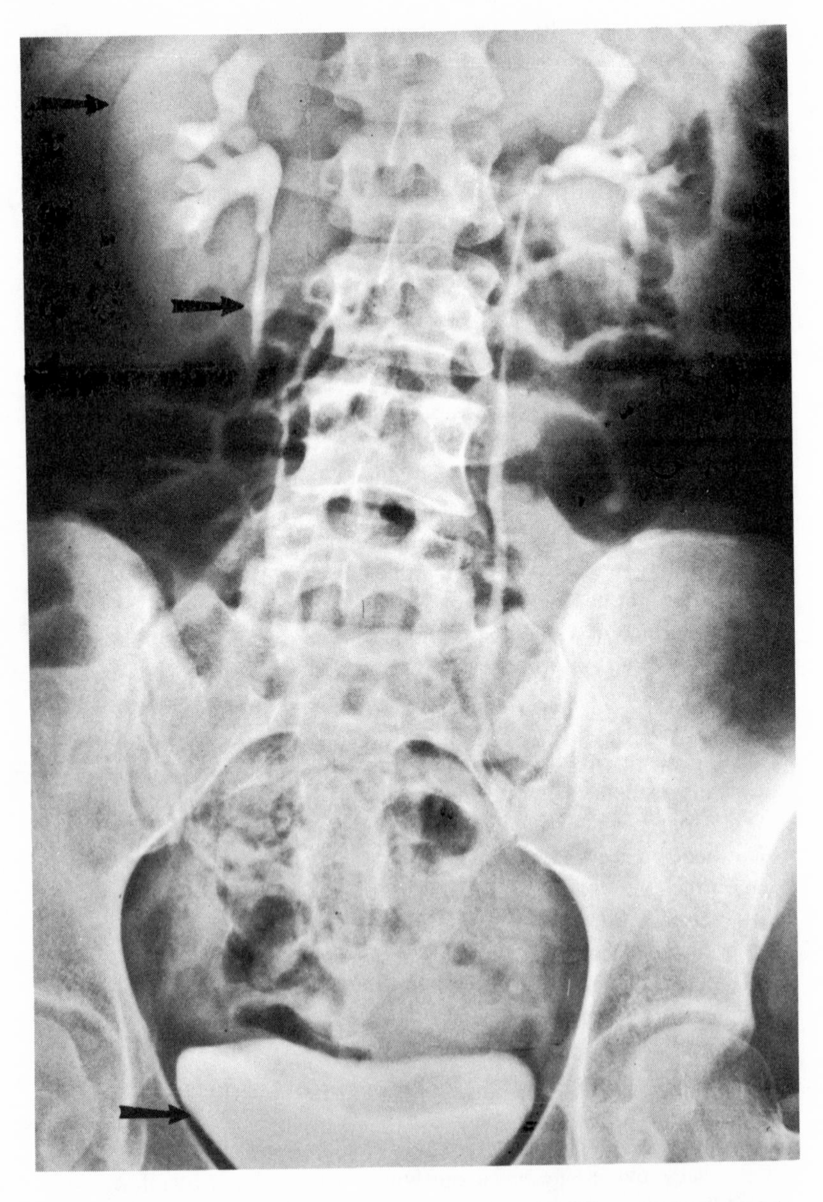

Figure 2-6. A normal excretory urogram showing the kidneys, the ureters, and the bladder.

a vein on the forearm that will concentrate in the kidneys and appear opaque against the dark background on the X ray (Fig. 2-6). The entire urinary system is seen on the films, and any abnormalities of the structure of the kidneys, ureters, bladder, and urethra can be clearly seen. Unfortunately, the intravenous substance that is injected into the vein may occasionally cause an allergic type of reaction, even an occasional fatal reaction. It is impossible to predict ahead of time which individuals will have severe reactions to the injected material even in those patients who have previously had an allergic reaction. In those patients, the radiologist customarily avoids taking the chance and usually will not perform the study. A new nonionic material is now available that has decreased the incidence of severe reactions and can be used in patients with a history of multiple allergies or reaction to previous urograms. Some patients may also be treated with cortisone derivatives (steroids) or with antihistamines as a protection against possible reaction to the material, but whether this offers any real protection is a subject of great controversy. There are several studies suggesting that a major risk factor for severe reaction is patient fear and anxiety.

Although the excretory urogram is of great value in the diagnosis of many urinary conditions, its value in diagnosis of obstructive BPH is somewhat limited and many urologists (the author included) do not recommend this test in the evaluation of a patient with symptoms of BPH, unless the patient has blood in the urine.

Ultrasound Examination

Ultrasound (also known as echography or sonogram) uses high-frequency sound waves to examine parts of the body. The abdominal ultrasound examination is a simple, noninvasive, and painless test. A small scanner is placed on the abdomen over the area of the kidneys. The scanner transmits sound waves that are electronically processed to form a fairly detailed picture on a television screen (Fig. 2-7), and the physician can check the kidneys for the presence of obstruction, tumors, stones, and other kidney problems.

The bladder can also be checked for residual urine with the ultrasound equipment. The patient is asked to empty his bladder, and then the ultrasound probe is placed on the lower part of the abdomen over the bladder area. An image of the bladder appears on the television screen

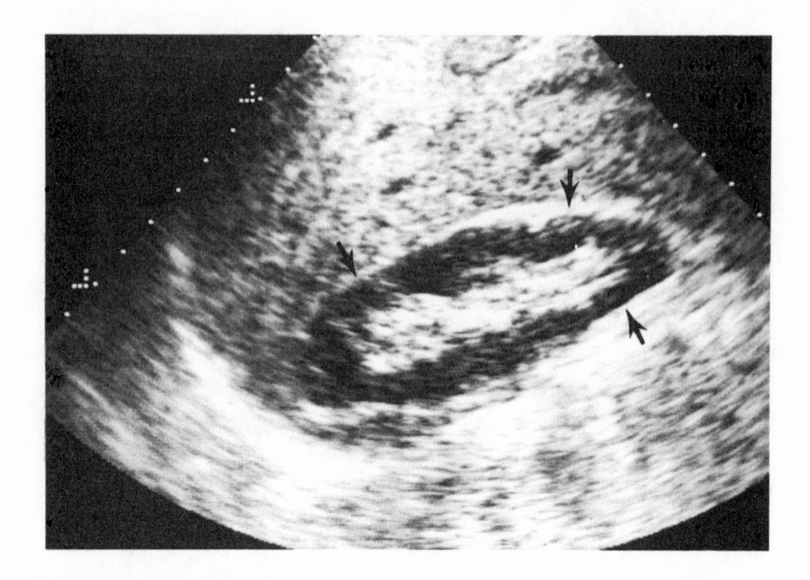

Figure 2-7. A normal ultrasound of the kidney. The kidney is outlined by the arrows.

and one can measure the approximate amount of residual urine left in the bladder after voiding. Otherwise, the residual urine is checked by inserting a catheter through the urethra into the bladder and measuring the volume as it drains into a container. This procedure is not only uncomfortable but can irritate the tissues, making the condition even worse. For examination of the prostate, a transrectal probe (Fig. 2-8) is inserted into the rectum and an image of the prostate appears on the television screen. This examination shows the size and shape of the prostate, but its most valuable use is in identifying possible prostate tumors and their location in the prostate.

Cystoscopy

Cystoscopy is the internal visual examination of the bladder and urethra. It is done using a pencil-thick hollow instrument that is either rigid or flexible (Fig. 2-9). A light exiting the end of the instrument illuminates the interior of the bladder and urethra, which can be examined through a viewing lens built into the instrument. This procedure is

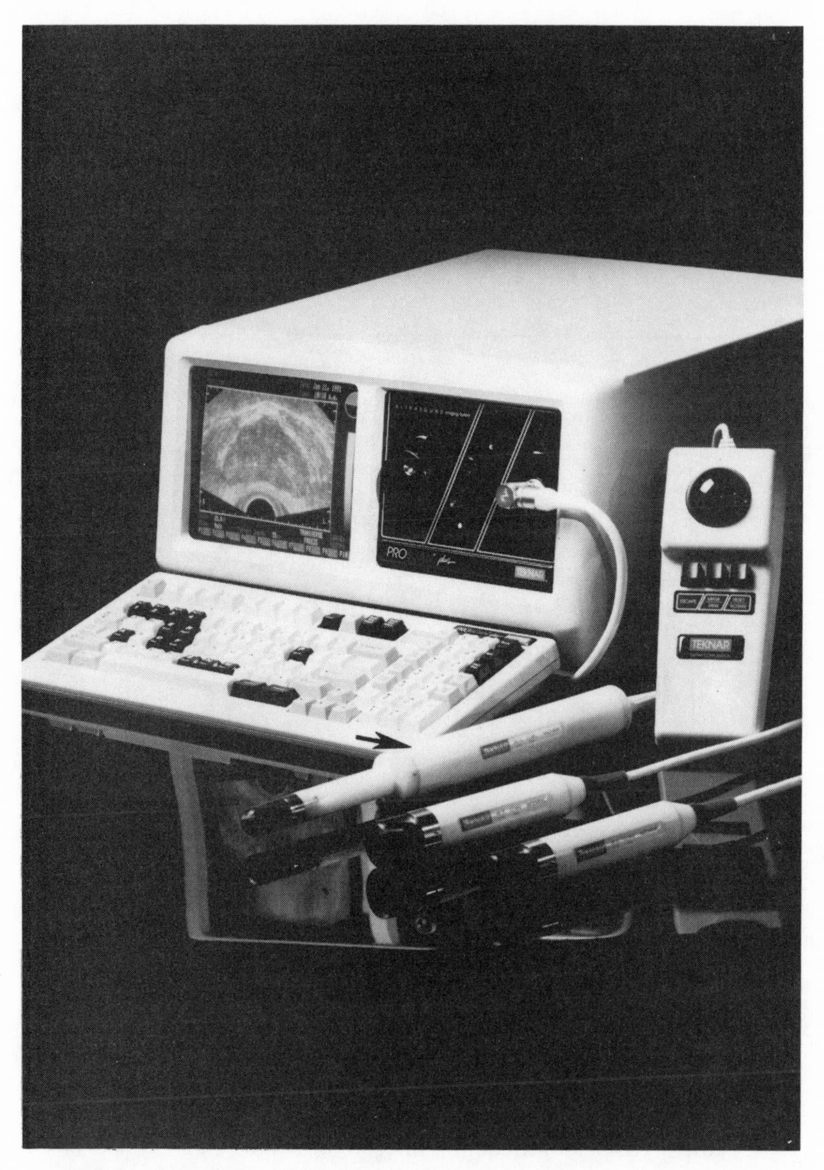

Figure 2-8. Ultrasound equipment. An image of the prostate can be seen on the television screen. The arrow points at a transrectal probe that is used to perform prostate ultrasound. (*Courtesy Teknar, Inc.*)

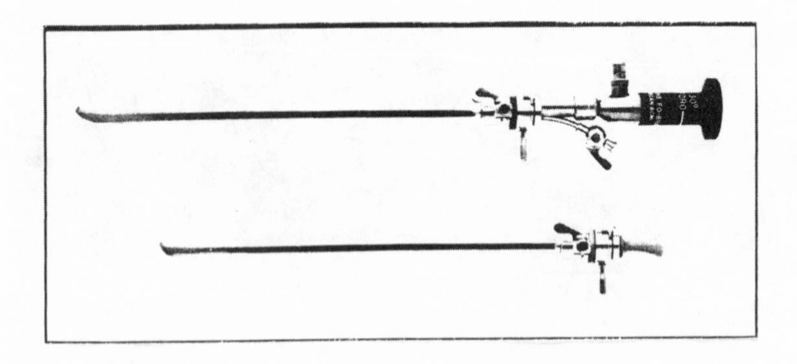

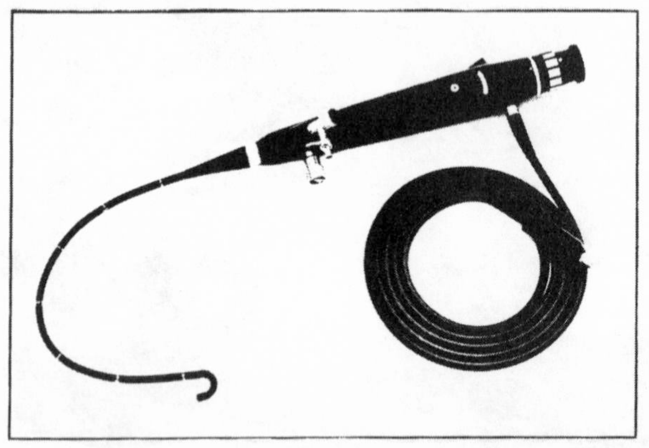

Figure 2-9. A rigid cystoscope (above) and a flexible cystoscope (below), for the internal visual examination of the bladder and urethra. (*Courtesy ACMI*)

frequently done in the urologist's office, after an anesthetic gel is instilled into the urethra through the opening in the penis. Done properly, cystoscopy should not be painful. By using a cystoscope, the urologist is able to see the interior of the bladder and prostatic urethra, and he can evaluate and assess the degree of obstruction in the prostatic urethra, estimate the size of the prostate, and check for other possible problems, such as bladder tumors, diveritcula, or stones.

Cystoscopy is seldom required in cases of simple BPH. It is absolutely necessary when blood is present in the urine. It is also helpful in determining the type of operation that the urologist would choose should surgery be indicated. This test is almost exclusively the domain of urologists and is one of the most useful tests in the field of urology.

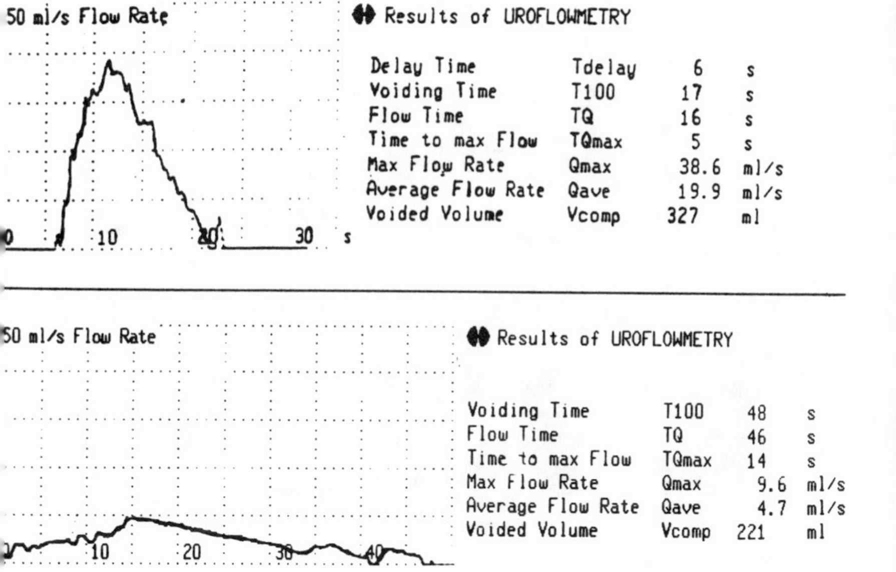

Figure 2-10. Uroflowmetry printout of a normal man (above) and that of a man with obstructive BPH (below).

Uroflowmetry

This is a simple and noninvasive test that determines the urinary flow rate. With BPH, the urinary stream becomes smaller as the disease progresses. An objective measure of how obstructed the prostatic urethra may be can be obtained by measuring the flow rate of the urinary stream that flows through it. The patient is asked to drink fluids until his bladder has reached its full capacity, and then is asked to void in a special container connected to an electronic instrument that prints out a graphic of the flow pattern and records the maximum peak flow and the amount of voided urine (Fig. 2-10). This simple test is very useful in evaluating the degree of obstruction present and the response to treatment.

Bladder Catheterization

Bladder catheterization is the act of passing a small hollow, flexible tube into the bladder through the urethra. One type of catheterization is

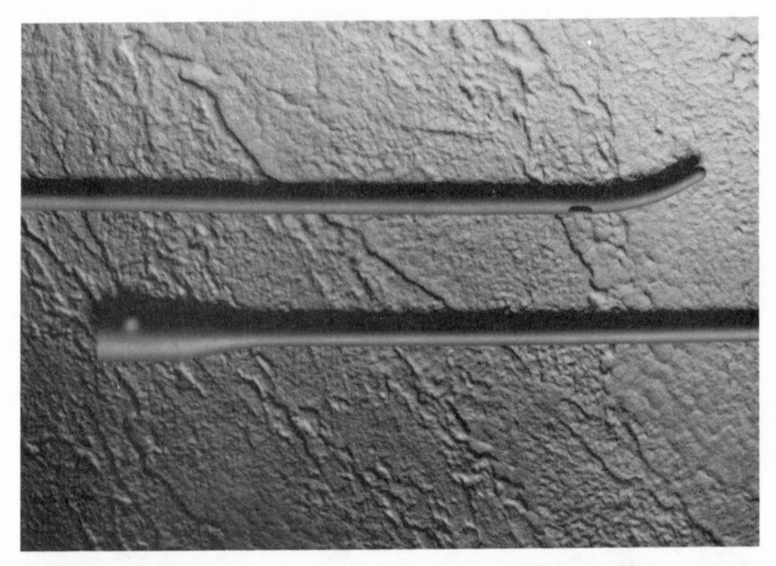

Figure 2-11. Straight catheter used for an ''in-and-out'' catheterization. (*Courtesy Bard Company*)

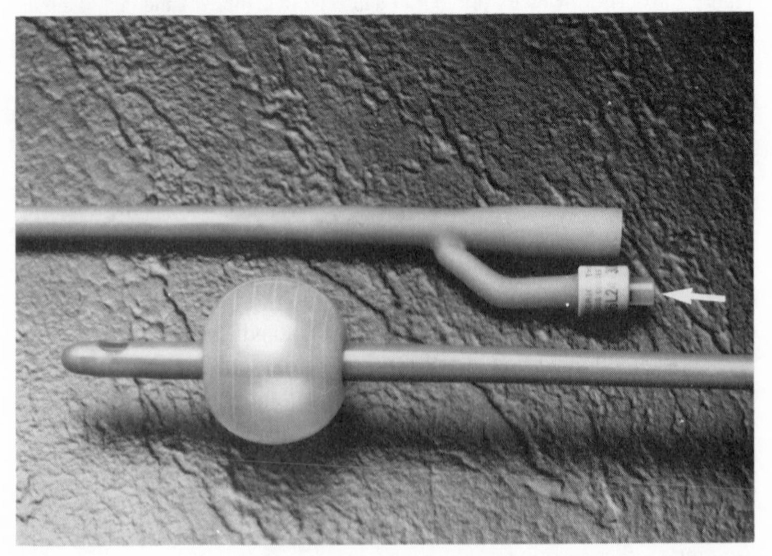

Figure 2-12. A Foley catheter, used when the catheter is to be in the bladder for a period of time. The arrow points to the sidearm on the catheter, through which water is injected to inflate the balloon at the end of the catheter. (*Courtesy the Bard Company*)

the ''in-and-out'' approach, in which the catheter (Fig. 2-11) is passed into the bladder for a very brief period of time, and then removed as in checking for residual urine or instilling solutions or medications into the bladder. This procedure is performed intermittently several times a day in patients who are unable to empty their bladders because of nerve deficiency, such as those who have suffered spinal injuries or strokes.

The second type of catheterization is done with a special catheter that can stay in the bladder for days or weeks at a time. Known as the **Foley catheter**, it has a balloon or bag at the tip that is inflated with water through a small channel. Once the balloon is inflated (Fig. 2-12), it prevents the catheter from slipping out accidentally. This is the type of catheter used after any surgical procedure to treat obstructive BPH. It is generally made of a flexible material such as rubber, latex, or other plastic.

CHAPTER 3

Treatment of Obstructive BPH

Standard Treatment Options

Nearly a century after the introduction of surgery for the treatment of obstructive BPH, surgery still remained the only possible option. However, surgery is now being challenged by a variety of alternative options that have emerged in recent years. Numerous drugs have been tested, balloon dilators have become available, and mechanical and thermal devices are under serious investigation.

At this time, it is important to mention that not all men who have symptoms of obstructive BPH need treatment; symptoms have been known to fluctuate over time and periods of spontaneous improvement in voiding symptoms have been frequently observed. Patients often show significant improvement in symptoms without any changes in objective obstructive findings such as flow rate, the amount of residual urine, or other similar parameters. This lack of correlation between patient symptoms, gland size, flow rates, and residual urine makes it difficult to establish standardized criteria for elective treatment. Each case has to be considered individually.

As of this writing, surgery continues to be the most effective treatment, but those cases in which the obstruction is not severe can often be managed successfully with drugs and adequate observation. The indications for treatment of symptomatic BPH can be of a medical or social nature.

Medical Indications

In some cases, surgery is mandatory and should be performed as soon as possible. Surgery is clearly indicated when the patient is completely unable to void, when large stones have developed in the bladder, when multiple bladder infections have resulted, repeated troublesome bleeding from the prostate has occurred, or when the obstruction is such that there is already kidney failure. For patients not having such severe conditions, management is less clear.

Social Indications

In some cases the severity of the symptoms may be such that it is the patient who decides treatment is necessary. The urinary frequency may be intolerable, urinary leakage may be embarrassing, or he may be tired of having to strain to urinate and of having no satisfaction with voiding. In some cases, urinary frequency causes the patient to change his lifestyle by avoiding situations that would make it difficult for him to urinate every hour or even more frequently. In these cases the patient often demands that something be done immediately.

In this chapter, we will discuss watchful waiting and various conventional surgical interventions being used today, as well as their side effects and complications. In Chapter 4, we will discuss current alternatives and treatments for obstructive BPH that are under investigation.

TREATMENT OF OBSTRUCTIVE BPH
Standard Options

- I. Watchful Waiting
- II. Surgery
  - A. Open Prostatectomy
    - 1. Suprapubic
    - 2. Retropubic
    - 3. Perineal
  - B. Transurethral: TURP
- III. Current Alternatives to Conventional Prostatectomy
  - A. Transurethal incision of the prostate (TUIP)
  - B. Balloon dilatation of the prostate (Uroplasty)
  - C. Visual Laser Prostatectomy

D. Medical treatment
1. Relaxing the prostate
2. Reducing the size of the prostate

IV. Treatment Under Investigation
A. Hormonal Manipulation
B. Transurethral Laser Induced Prostatectomy (TULIP)
C. Hypothermia
D. Prostate Stents

I. WATCHFUL WAITING

The man who has only mild symptoms of obstructive BPH and no significant findings to suggest severe obstruction can be safely placed on observation, with periodic testing of urinary flow rate and determination of residual urine. It is estimated that about 30 percent of patients under observation alone will experience spontaneous improvement of their obstructive symptoms. Many patients do not show a worsening of their symptoms and can go for years without having any significant problem.

II. SURGERY

The operation to correct obstruction due to BPH is called **prostatectomy**. In prostatectomy, only the part of the gland that is causing obstruction is removed, so that the surgical capsule or "true" prostate remains. The anatomy of an enlarged prostate is quite different from that of a normal prostate. When BPH develops the enlarged prostate consists of the periurethral benign growth, or adenoma, the remaining "normal prostate" and the external capsule or shell (Fig. 3-1). The normal prostate has often been compressed by the expanding adenoma. In explaining prostatectomy to my patients, I frequently compare the enlarged gland to an orange. The operation removes the meat, leaving the peel or external shell. The meat in the orange would correspond to the adenoma or the part of the gland that is causing the obstruction. The peel of the orange would correspond to the compressed normal prostate and capsule. When the obstructive adenoma is removed, the prostatic urethra contained within the adenoma is removed as well (Fig. 3-2).

The term prostatectomy is a misnomer, since by definition it means the removal of the prostate, and in this procedure only the adenoma or the part of the prostate that is causing the obstruction is removed. A more appropriate term would be prostate adenomectomy. However, the

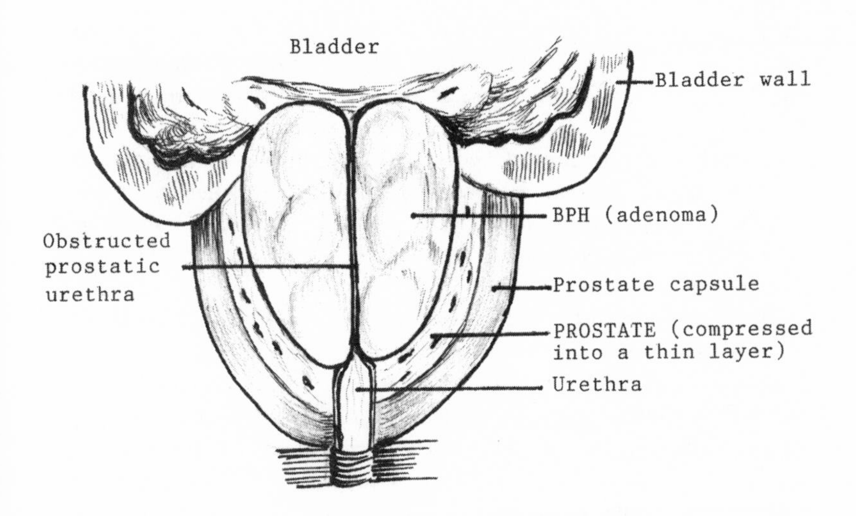

Figure 3-1. Prostate showing markedly obstructed BPH.

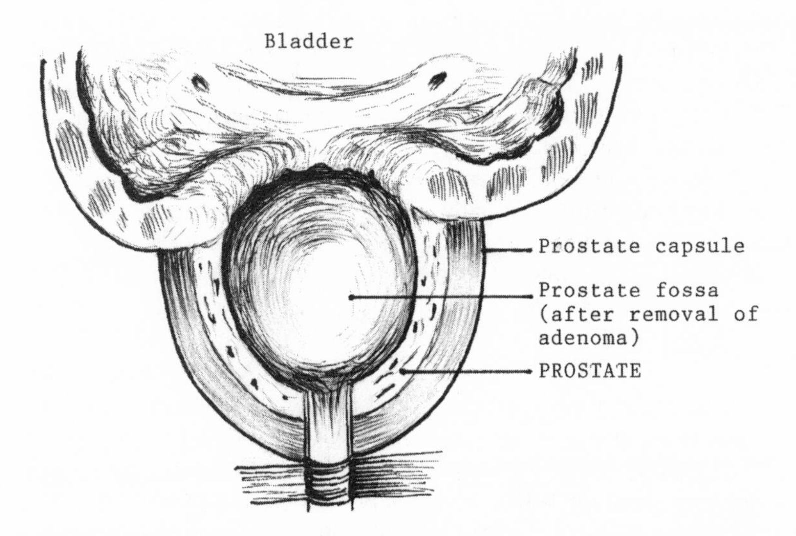

Figure 3-2. When the obstructive adenoma is removed, a cavity known as the prostate fossa is left. The prostatic urethra contained within the adenoma is removed as well.

term "prostatectomy" continues to be used, although only with the understanding that the entire prostate is not removed. When the entire gland is removed, as in the case of prostate cancer, the term **radical prostatectomy** is used.

Many men become confused when the physician checks their prostate after they have undergone prostatectomy for BPH. They need to be told that they still have part of the prostate and that they still have the same chance of developing cancer of the prostate as anyone else, and that therefore they should have it checked annually.

There are two types of prostatectomy to treat BPH: **open prostatectomy**, in which the surgeon makes an incision in the skin to remove the obstructive part of the prostate, and **transurethral prostatectomy**, which is performed entirely through the urethra using an instrument similar to the cystoscope, known as a resectoscope. The transurethral approach is by far the most commonly used and is also the least painful and least disturbing for the patient. This approach requires much more surgical skill than any of the open surgical procedures.

A. Open Prostatectomy. There are three common surgical approaches for open prostatectomy: suprapubic, retropubic, and perineal. The suprapubic and retropubic approaches require an incision in the lower part of the abdomen. The term "pubic" refers to the pubic bone (the bone situated just over the base of the penis). The perineal approach is performed through an incision in the area between the scrotum and the rectum, the perineum.

1. Suprapubic Prostatectomy. To perform a suprapubic prostatectomy, the surgeon usually makes a vertical incision in the lower part of the abdomen—from just below the navel to the pubic bone. Occasionally, the urologist chooses to make a transverse low abdominal incision (Fig. 3-3). The incision is extended through the layers of the abdominal wall—until the bladder is exposed. The bladder is then opened and the BPH or prostate adenoma is removed through the open bladder (Fig. 3-4). Generally, two catheters are left in the bladder, one through the urethra and the other through a small opening made in the wall of the bladder and anterior or abdominal wall. Credit for developing this prostate operation by making it simple, safe, and effective goes to Sir Peter Freyer of St. Peter's Hospital in London. Freyer's operation was described in 1901.

2. Retropubic Prostatectomy. Retropubic prostatectomy is the most recently developed of the four present-day traditional surgical approaches to the prostate. Suprapubic prostatectomy had been the

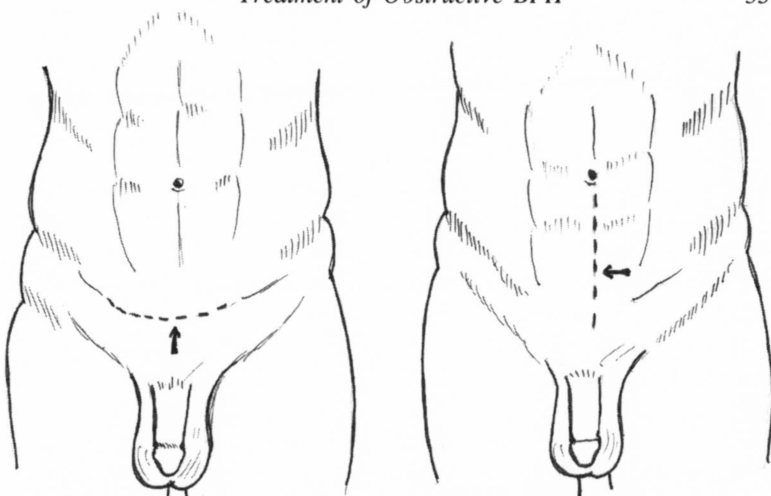

Figure 3-3. The place in the lower abdomen where the incision is made for prostatectomy.

standard approach for some forty years until an Irish surgeon, Terrance Millen, described his retropubic prostatectomy in 1945. This operation is also performed through an incision in the lower part of the abdomen, but the bladder is not opened, as in the case of the suprapubic prostatectomy. An incision is made directly through the prostate capsule and the adenoma is removed through the incision (Fig. 3-5). Only one catheter is left in the bladder through the urethra in this operation. The advantages of the retropubic approach are that it permits excellent exposure of the prostate and greatly facilitates control of bleeding after the obstructive tissue has been removed.

3. Perineal Prostatectomy. In this surgical approach an incision is made in the perineum, the area between the scrotum and the anus (Fig. 3-6). This is by far the oldest of the three types of surgical exposure for treatment of BPH. This approach was very popular for many years, but at present it is rarely performed, mainly because it produces a higher incidence of impotence postoperatively than any of the other methods. This is presumably because of injury to the nerves that control erection, that are exposed to possible damage in this approach.

B. Transurethral Resection of the Prostate (TURP). This operation is by far the procedure most commonly used today to treat patients with obstructive BPH. Approximately 400,000 transurethral prostatectomies (TURPs) are performed in the United States each year.

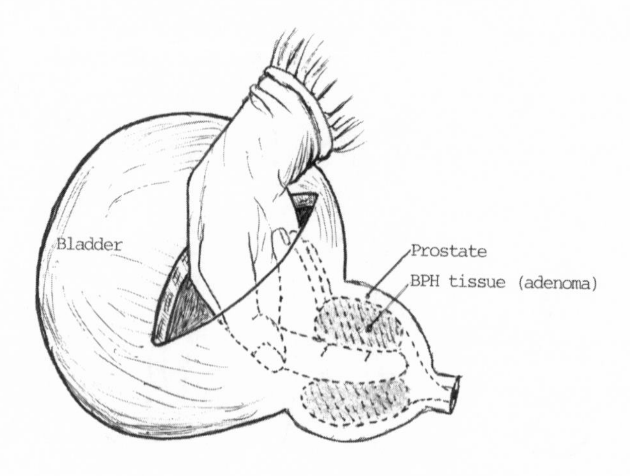

Figure 3-4. A suprapubic prostatectomy. An incision has been made through the bladder for removal of the BPH tissue (adenoma).

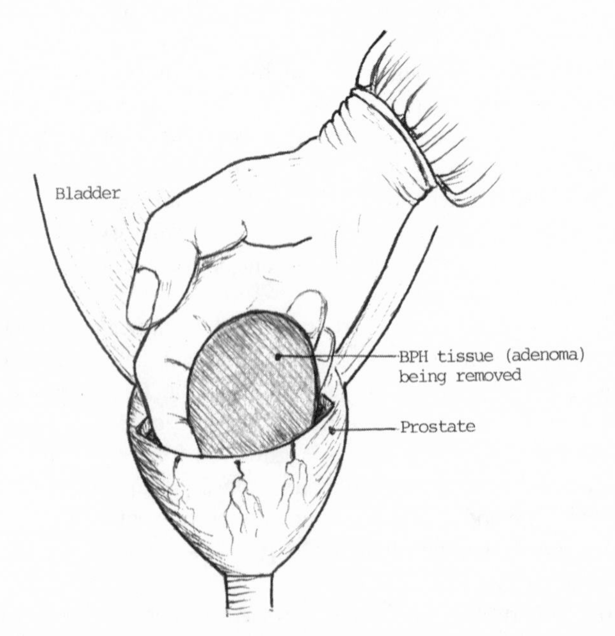

Figure 3-5. A retropubic prostatectomy. In this case the incision is made not through the bladder but through the prostate capsule for removal of BPH tissue (adenoma).

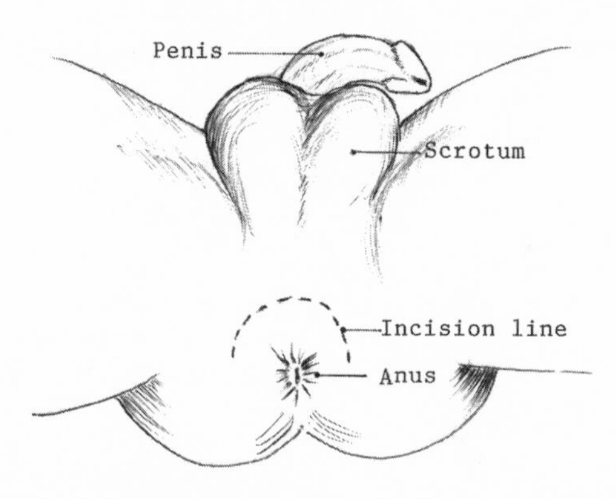

Figure 3-6. The perineal area. The incision line indicates where the incision for perineal prostatectomy is made.

The entire operation is performed through the urethra, using a well-lubricated instrument similar to the cystoscope, called the resectoscope (Fig. 3-7). A small wire loop at the end of the resectoscope is connected to an electric source, and when electricity is activated the wire loop cuts through the obstructive tissue as it is moved back and forth. At the end of the procedure all the prostate chips are evacuated and a Foley catheter is placed in the bladder through the urethra. The technique and instrumentation used in this procedure have been polished and refined over the years, to make TURP today an excellent, successful, and safe surgical procedure comparable to open surgery in results, but with the advantage that no incision is necessary.

Choosing the Right Operation

TURP is an excellent procedure and, as mentioned above, is by far the most commonly used. This procedure is clearly the operation of choice to treat most cases of obstructive BPH whenever the prostate is not extremely large. There are certain groups of patients for whom the transurethral approach is not suitable and who must undergo an open prostatectomy. When the prostate gland is extremely large, an open operation may be required for two reasons: first, it takes longer to remove tissue by TURP in these cases, and the surgeon may be reluctant to carry out a very long operation, especially in an elderly patient who has other medical problems; and second, the prostatic urethra may be so

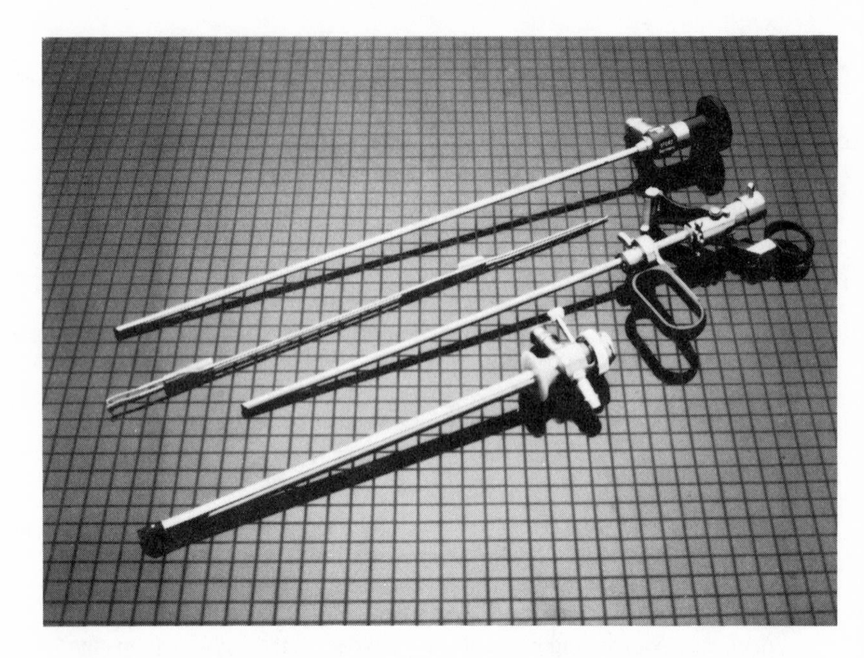

Figure 3-7. Above: Different components of one of the available resectoscopes used in transurethral resection of the prostate (TURP). (*Courtesy Karl Storz*) Below: Transurethral resection of the prostate being performed with a resectoscope. The surgeon is cutting away small fragments of obstructive prostate tissue.

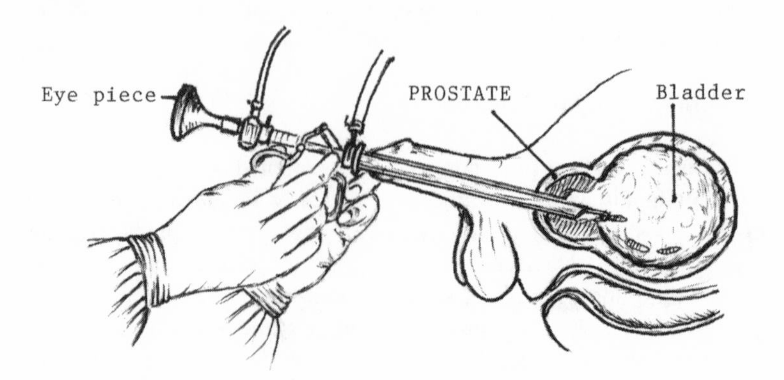

long that it is difficult to reach the neck of the bladder with the resectoscope. Patients who have very narrow urethras or severe strictures may also require the open procedure to avoid trauma to the urethra that might result in further urethral scarring.

Another group of patients who may require open surgery are those who have large bladder stones or large bladder diverticula which require surgical removal. This can be performed at the same time of the open prostatectomy and through the same incision. Many patients who have some osteoarthritis of the hip joints may also require an open operation, because the stiffness of the joints makes it impossible to position the patient correctly for TURP (with his knees elevated and separated).

Limitations and Complications of Prostatectomy for BPH

Unfortunately, no surgical procedures, even minor operations, are exempted from complications, and prostatectomy, being a major surgical procedure, is associated with several side effects and possible complications. The following are the most common of them:

- Retrograde ejaculation
- Postoperative bleeding
- Impotence
- Incontinence
- Contracture of the bladder neck
- Urethral stricture
- Epididymitis
- TUR Syndrome

Retrograde Ejaculation

Rather than a complication, retrograde ejaculation is a side effect of prostatectomy. Normal ejaculation is antigrade—that is, semen flows through the urethra from the prostate to the outside. The semen cannot go into the bladder through the neck of the bladder because at the time of ejaculation the neck of the bladder closes. Occasionally after prostatectomy, the neck of the bladder may lose its ability to contract and close, so that when semen enters the urethra it follows the path of least resistance, and rather than going through a long narrow channel (the urethra), it goes through the open bladder neck into the bladder. This is known as retrograde ejaculation. The semen will mix with the urine in the bladder and is evacuated in the next voiding. Patients with this condition will continue to experience climax, but since no semen comes out through the urethra during orgasm, men have a "dry climax." Retrograde ejaculation sometimes is not completely "dry" so that some semen is ejaculated.

In a select group of patients, it is possible to leave the neck of the bladder intact, particularly during TURP, to preserve normal ejaculation. When retrograde ejaculation occurs, the sensation of orgasm is still present, although some men say they feel that the sensation is not quite the same as before surgery. In cases where men are still interested in fathering children, an alternative procedure should be considered.

Postoperative Bleeding

As a general rule, bleeding, which may occur during the operation, is controlled by the end of the operation and the bleeding that occurs during the first day or two after surgery is minimal. During surgery, it is not possible to control all bleeding vessels, and this accounts for the mild bleeding that occurs in the immediate postoperative period. Many times the gradual dissolution of a clot in the bladder is the cause of postoperative bleeding—generous bladder irrigation will help.

During TURP, the surgeon cauterizes bleeding blood vessels with the same instrument used to remove the prostatic tissue. This leads to scab formation. By the time the scab falls off, a few weeks after surgery, the vessels will have healed. Occasionally, when the scab peels, the patient may have some renewed bleeding, which in most instances will stop spontaneously. However, in some cases the bleeding may be severe enough to necessitate blood transfusions or to cause clot retention, often resulting in readmission to the hospital for treatment.

Impotence

The possibility of impotence after prostate surgery is worrisome to many patients. The cause of impotence following prostate surgery is not clear and there is no convincing reason why some patients become impotent. Certainly nothing is done during prostatectomy that should alter libido or prevent a man from obtaining an erection. The tissue removed is well within the prostate and cannot damage the nerves that control erections, which are outside the capsule. The reported rate of postoperative impotence in males who were functioning normally prior to surgery ranges from 5 to 25 percent. Most urologists would agree that less than 10 percent is a realistic rate.

Several investigations have indicated that there are risk factors that may enhance the occurrence of impotence after surgery, mainly poor erection preoperatively, and advanced age. The highest incidence of impotence is reported in older patients and in those with a history of cardiovascular disease. It is a known fact that any surgical procedure performed on elderly men can precipitate impotence, or at least a lack of interest in sex, but the exact cause is not clear. It can be said, however, that patients who have a stable and satisfying sexual relationship prior to surgery will most likely have no postoperative problem. There are even occasional cases in which patients report improvement in their sex life after surgery. This may be attributed to the fact that they generally feel better not being under the constant stress caused by severe symptoms of prostate obstruction.

Incontinence

Perhaps the most distressing and unpleasant complication of prostatectomy is incontinence, where the man loses the ability to control his urine. A small proportion of patients become incontinent, but fortunately this problem is temporary in the great majority of cases. Within six months nearly all patients have good control. A few patients, however, become permanently incontinent, requiring drug therapy or surgery to correct their problem. Currently in the United States, it is estimated that less than 1 percent of the male population will become incontinent after surgery to the point where treatment is necessary. The most popular surgical procedure to treat incontinence is the use of an artificial sphincter. This sphincter, implanted surgically around the urethra next to the true sphincter, is a circular cuff connected to a pump mechanism (Fig. 3-8) buried in the upper part of the scrotum that the patient may control by pressing a button when he wants to urinate.

Contracture of the Bladder Neck

This is a rare but troublesome complication of any prostatectomy. The open surface of the bladder neck heals after surgery by scarring, and

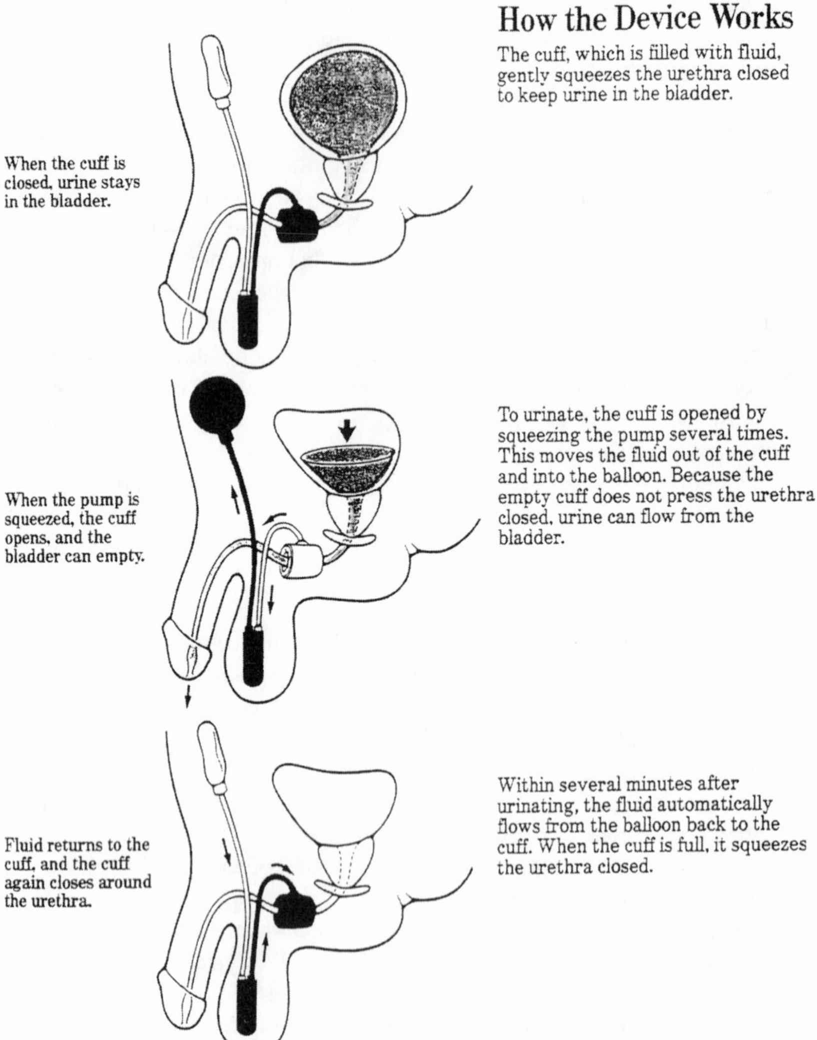

How the Device Works

The cuff, which is filled with fluid, gently squeezes the urethra closed to keep urine in the bladder.

When the cuff is closed, urine stays in the bladder.

To urinate, the cuff is opened by squeezing the pump several times. This moves the fluid out of the cuff and into the balloon. Because the empty cuff does not press the urethra closed, urine can flow from the bladder.

When the pump is squeezed, the cuff opens, and the bladder can empty.

Within several minutes after urinating, the fluid automatically flows from the balloon back to the cuff. When the cuff is full, it squeezes the urethra closed.

Fluid returns to the cuff, and the cuff again closes around the urethra.

Figure 3-8. An artificial sphincter in place. The entire device is placed inside the body, so nothing can be seen from the outside. (*Diagram courtesy American Medical Systems*)

when the scarring is severe, it may cause the neck of the bladder to contract and become obstructive. The resulting small bladder neck frequently causes more obstruction and more symptoms than the original prostate obstruction. This problem can usually be corrected easily and successfully with either dilatation or transurethral incision of the vesical neck.

Urethral Stricture

Urethral stricture means narrowing of some part of the urethra and is, as in the case of contracture of the bladder neck, generally caused by scarring of the urethra due to urethral trauma. They are more common following a TURP. The symptoms can be more alarming than those caused by the original prostate obstruction. In TURP, the trauma to the urethra may be caused by using a resectoscope too large for the size of the urethra, or, more likely, by poor lubrication of the instrument. When strictures occur, they can be treated by stretching (dilating) the urethra periodically with urethral dilators, a relatively simple office procedure. Occasionally, transurethral incision through the scar, a procedure called visual urethrotomy, may be necessary. Strictures occur in approximately 3 percent of patients who undergo TURP. It happens even less frequently after open prostatectomy.

Epididymitis

This is an unpleasant but now very rare complication of prostate surgery probably because of the more frequent routine use of antibiotics and the use of a catheter for a shorter period of time after surgery. The most common symptoms are generally pain and swelling of one or both testes caused by inflammation and infection of the epididymis, a tube-like structure that wraps around one side of the testis. It presumably occurs because infection from the prostate has spread through the vas deferens to the epididymis. It seems to occur more commonly when the prostate has been infected just prior to prostate surgery or when a catheter has been in the bladder for some time prior to surgery. The treatment of this condition generally includes bed rest, antibiotics, ice applied locally, painkillers, and in some cases the use of an athletic supporter. It usually subsides within a few days with treatment.

TUR Syndrome

This is a rare complication of TURP, which generally becomes manifested during or at the end of the operation. It is apparently caused by reabsorption into the bloodstream of the special fluid used for irrigation during the operation. The fact that the blood becomes diluted and the sodium level drops considerably seems to be the basis of the syndrome, which is an alteration of the cardiovascular, renal, and neurological functions. The vital signs show significant alteration, and several neurological symptoms develop, such as confusion, irritability, convulsions, and sometimes coma and kidney failure. All urologists are very much aware of this possibility, and with proper technique it can be avoided. Fortunately, it rarely occurs at present. Treatment is based on administration of both diuretics and sodium infusion.

CHAPTER 4

Treatment of Obstructive BPH

Current Alternatives and Treatments Under Investigation

III. CURRENT ALTERNATIVES TO CONVENTIONAL PROSTATECTOMY.

A. TRANSURETHRAL INCISION OF THE PROSTATE (TUIP). This procedure is an excellent alternative to TURP for relief of symptoms of BPH. It is performed mostly on patients who have small obstructive glands. One or two incisions are made through the bladder neck and through the entire length of the prostate. TUIP usually results in significant improvement of obstructive symptoms, improvement in urinary peak flow rates, and residual urine equal to TURP. Over 80 percent of patients treated with TUIP will remain able to ejaculate normally. Some patients, however, will need TURP if obstructive symptoms persist. A need for subsequent TURP has been reported in from 1.5 to 13 percent of patients.

TUIP is a procedure of short duration that produces a minimal loss of blood. It can be performed under spinal epidural or general anesthesia. In a selected group of patients, such as older patients with serious diseases, it would be more advantageous to attempt to carry out this procedure under local anesthesia.

The Advantages of TUIP Over TURP:

- It is a simpler and shorter procedure
- It can be done under local anesthesia with intravenous sedation
- The procedure does not always require hospitalization
- Blood loss is significantly reduced
- It does not result in impotence
- Retrograde ejaculation occurs only in less than 16 percent (literature average) of cases
- There is a shorter convalescence and recovery period

The Disadvantages of TUIP:

- No tissue is removed for microscopic examination
- TUIP is not suitable for large glands (it is recommended only for small glands)
- It is not effective in all cases and some patients may later require TURP

Most urologists agree that TUIP is largely underutilized and should be considered in patients who are sexually active, who have symptoms of prostate obstruction, and who have small glands.

B. Balloon Dilatation of the Prostate (Uroplasty). Many younger patients who are troubled by symptoms of urinary flow obstruction seek alternatives to prostatectomy in an effort to avoid the risk of retrograde ejaculation or impotence. With such patients, balloon dilatation of the prostate may play a short-term role. The effect of balloon dilatation, however, is not permanent, and the procedure may have to be repeated in six months.

Patients who have only a limited life expectancy, or who are medically unfit for longer surgical procedures, require a simpler and more effective means of relieving retention or symptoms of obstruction. It is for this group of patients that this procedure is most beneficial. The stretching of the prostate capsule and compacting of the prostate tissue results in a stretching and widening of the prostatic urethra and improved urine flow.

Balloon dilatation is an easy procedure to perform and is done under local anesthesia in most instances. The complication rate is low and it is performed on an outpatient basis. It is not effective for very large glands or when an enlarged median lobe is present. Balloon dilatation is performed after a catheter has been passed into the urethra (Fig. 4-1). A balloon located at the end of the catheter is inflated for a period of ten to

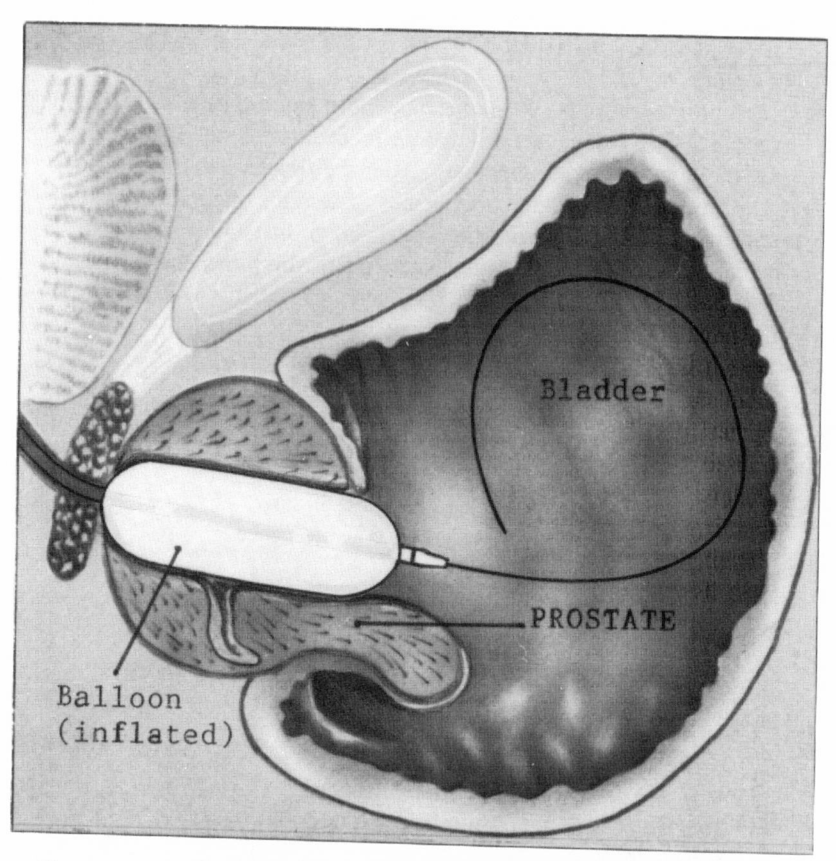

Figure 4-1. A balloon dilatation of the prostate being performed. An inflatable balloon has been placed inside the prostatic urethra. (*Courtesy Macrovesive*)

fifteen minutes. The exact mechanism by which this procedure works is not clearly understood, but pressure is exerted on the prostate tissue, compressing it and stretching the prostate capsule. The final result seems to be the decompression of the prostatic urethra.

The concept of dilatation of the prostatic urethra for the purpose of relieving prostate obstruction is not new. As early as 1844, a metallic dilator was designed with the intention of disrupting and dilating the prostatic urethra and vesical neck. The results, however, were not very encouraging, and interest in this procedure declined. It was not until balloons were designed to dilate obstructed blood vessels in the late

1970s that the first balloon dilatation of the prostate gland was attempted.

Preliminary results of trials comparing balloon dilatation with conventional TURP demonstrated that the procedures produced comparable results in reduction of symptoms. After the first twelve months, however, recurrence of symptoms began to develop, and recent reports indicate that forty-eight months after balloon dilatation, only about 13 percent of patients still show benefit from this procedure. Its main drawback appears to be its short effect, and patients who select this form of therapy need to be aware of this.

The Advantages of Balloon Dilatation Over Conventional TURP:

- It is much simpler to perform
- Hospitalization may not be necessary
- It can be performed under local anesthesia
- There is a shorter recovery and convalescence
- It is less expensive
- It does not cause impotence
- There is a very low complication rate
- Retrograde ejaculation generally does not occur

The Disadvantages of Balloon Dilatation:

- The effect is unpredictable
- It is only effective in smaller prostates
- The effect is of short duration, and the procedure may need to be repeated
- No tissue is removed for microscopic examination

C. VISUAL LASER PROSTATECTOMY. One alternative to the traditional TURP that is demonstrating significant benefits is the use of neodymium YAG (otherwise known as Nd:YAG) laser to perform the prostatectomy.

One of the advantages of laser energy over conventional TURP is that lasers cause coagulation of radiated tissue and associated blood vessels so that bleeding generally does not occur.

The Nd:YAG laser is a standard surgical laser in widespread use and already found in many hospital operating rooms. In performing visual prostatectomy, the surgeon employs a system that uses a flexible laser fiber that delivers high energy at a right angle to allow the application of energy directly perpendicular to the fiber.

To use this system, a regular rigid cystoscope is passed through the urethra into the bladder. The laser floor is passed through the cystoscope and several laser applications are made to all four quadrants of the prostatic urethra.

The surgical goal is to coagulate a sufficient depth of tissue so that, with sloughing, a cavity is produced.

Clinical trials to date have affirmed the overall safety of this system. In the short term (up to one year) its efficacy is comparable to standard TURP, both in terms of objective parameters and subjective symptom improvement. Although the results of this technology are excellent, the follow-up remains limited since it is a very new procedure.

Dr. Thomas Stamey, a renowned authority in urology, in a recent publication in the 1993 *Monographs in Urology* states that very soon even very large prostates will ultimately be treated by laser techniques, and that the procedure will replace conventional TURP.

The Advantages of Nd:YAG Are:

- The operation is very simple and takes very little time
- The operation can be done under epidural or spinal anesthesia
- Bleeding is uncommon
- It is an outpatient procedure
- The results are comparable to those of TURP
- Ejaculation is not affected as with TURP

The Disadvantages of Nd:YAG Are:

- A catheter is required for no less than four days
- No tissue is removed for microscopic examination

D. MEDICAL (NONSURGICAL) TREATMENT OF BPH. For centuries, attempts have been made to find a medical treatment that is satisfactory as an alternative to surgery for BPH. The development of an effective agent to treat symptoms of BPH would not only be of obvious benefit to patients who are poor risks for surgical treatment, but would have a considerable economic impact.

Over the past five years, the interest in nonsurgical therapy for BPH has escalated. The intensified search for alternatives to surgical treatment has been motivated by a scientific community committed to developing optional treatments for this common condition; by a federal government that is seeking to cut down on the significant expense of TURP for treatment of prostate enlargement in the Medicare population and to stem the rising costs of medical treatment imposed on the public; by powerful drug companies seeking to develop a competitive edge; and by the global trend to minimize invasive procedures. In addition, the urologic community has been concerned with the nature and severity of complications of prostatectomy and by the fact that not all patients who undergo this procedure have a satisfactory outcome. Approximately 15 percent of men will require a repeat operation within eight years after TURP.

Although TURP is likely to remain the most effective treatment of BPH for some time to come, the limitations of this procedure justify the search for alternative nonsurgical treatments.

BPH is a disease characterized by spontaneous improvement, and it is thus not surprising that in many studies improvement is noticed in both treated and placebo (sugar-pill) controls after a short period of time. This makes evaluation of the effect of the treatment very difficult.

In searching for a medical treatment, the mechanism of obstruction in BPH has to be understood. The mechanism by which the enlarged prostate restricts the bladder outflow is thought to be due to:

1—A mechanical "static effect" caused by the bulk of the prostate mass, and
2—A "dynamic" muscular component resulting from stimulation of receptors in the prostate smooth muscle, and in the muscle of the neck of the bladder

The relevant importance of these two factors has been disputed. While some researchers feel that the bulk is what causes the obstruction, and therefore the obstructive symptoms, others feel that the muscular tone is just as important. After reviewing the literature on current research, one reaches the conclusion that the most effective nonsurgical treatment should be aimed at reducing both obstructive components: bulk and muscle tone. Treatment aimed at only one or the other will have a limited effect, whereas one that considers both of these elements should reduce both the size of the enlarged prostate and also the muscular tone, and will be much more effective.

1. Relaxing the Prostate. As the prostate enlarges, the contractibility of its smooth muscle is used inappropriately on the urethra,

thus clamping the flow of urine. The so-called alpha-adrenergic blockers are a category of drugs known to relax smooth muscle. These have been used to treat high blood pressure by relaxing the smooth muscle in the wall of the arteries. They have a similar effect on the smooth muscle of the prostate and bladder neck, and therefore reduce resistance to the flow of urine. Approximately 20 percent of the obstructive prostate enlargement is smooth muscle that has the capacity to contract.

At present, there are three alpha blockers available for clinical use, even though they are not approved by the Food and Drug Administration (FDA) for BPH. Prazosin (brand name Minipres) was introduced in 1977 as an antihypertensive agent. Several studies have shown benefit in patients with symptomatic BPH who have taken this medication. Another alpha blocker categorized as an antihypertensive agent is Terazosin (brand name Hytrin). The primary advantage of Terazosin over other commercially available alpha blockers is that its longer half-life allows for a once-daily dosing regimen usually taken at bedtime.

Several studies conducted in the United States and Europe suggest that Terazosin is effective in the control of symptoms associated with BPH. One recent multicenter study conducted in the United States, using once-daily administration of this drug, reported an overall urinary flow rate increase of 50 percent. There was a 67 percent improvement in symptom scores, and 35 percent improvement in irritative symptoms. The adverse reactions, which occurred in about 5 percent of patients, included headaches in about 10 percent of these cases, weakness in about 7 percent, and dizziness in about 14 percent. All adverse reactions disappeared upon termination of drug administration. Although the ideal alpha blocker for patients with symptoms of obstructive BPH has not been developed, data suggest that the alpha blockers available do ameliorate symptoms and may play a more significant role in the future.

The third alpha blocker available for clinical use is Doxazosin (brand name Cardura). The use of this drug has not been as extensive as the use of Prazosin in the treatment of obstructive BPH. Like the other two alpha blockers mentioned earlier, Doxazosin is primarily an antihypertensive agent.

At a recent meeting of the American Urological Association in San Antonio, Texas, several studies evaluating this drug in terms of safety, effect on obstructive systems of BPH, and effect on blood pressure were presented. Patients experienced a statistical, significant improvement in symptoms with treatment of Doxazosin, as well as improvements on flow rates. The effects on blood pressure in normotensive patients was not significant, and it appears that it provides a safe and satisfactory alternative to similar drugs.

2. Reducing the Size of the Prostate. In contrast to surgical castration, where the testes are removed, nonsurgical castration, or medical castration, tries to produce the same effect without surgery by blocking the function of the testicles. But the problem with medical castration, too, is the subsequent loss of sexual function, and for this reason, like surgical castration, this treatment has not been well accepted. Researchers learned that no hormonal treatment would be satisfactory if the treatment resulted in sexual malfunction.

5-Alpha Reductase Inhibitor Therapy—Finasteride (brand name Proscar), the most recent hormonal approach to treating BPH by reducing prostate size, has been based on the observation that BPH does not occur in individuals genetically deficient in an enzyme—5-alpha reductase. This is an enzyme that converts the male hormone testosterone (T) to dihydrotestosterone (DT). Testosterone is the male hormone that is responsible for libido and sexual function. Dihydrotestosterone is the predominant intracellular male hormone that acts on prostate growth. By blocking this enzyme, and therefore the production of dihydrotestosterone, testosterone levels continue to be normal and therefore libido and sexual function are not affected, but the lack of dihydrotestosterone will reduce prostate size.

A drug known as Finasteride (brand name Proscar) blocks the action of 5-alpha reductase and reduces circulating levels of dihydrotestosterone without lowering levels of testosterone. The Finasteride Study Group, which has participants from twenty-five medical centers in the United States and five in Canada, reported its findings after the first year of research with finasteride, in *The New England Journal of Medicine* issue of October 22, 1992. Of 297 patients who received 5 mg of finasteride daily, there was a 23 percent reduction in obstructive symptoms and 31 percent of the men had a significant increase in urinary flow rate. After twelve months of treatment, the patients showed also a decrease in the size of the prostate gland of 19 percent from baseline.

This drug also has an excellent safety profile. Proscar is generally well tolerated; adverse reactions have been for the most part mild and transient. The volume of ejaculation may be decreased in some patients during treatment; this decrease, however, does not appear to interfere with normal sexual function. The incidence of impotence in patients taking Proscar has been reported at 3.7 percent.

One of the drawbacks to the use of Proscar is that its use results in decrease of PSA. PSA (Prostate Specific Antigen) is a protein produced by the prostate gland, and elevated blood levels of this substance can be observed in men with cancer of the prostate (see Chapter 6). The reduction of PSA levels in men who are being treated with Proscar should be considered when they are evaluated for the possibility of prostate cancer. In addition, any sustained increase or lack of decrease in PSA levels while on Proscar should therefore be very carefully evaluated.

Another drawback to the use of Proscar is that although there is a regression in the size of the enlarged prostate, fewer than 30 percent of patients treated experience improvement in symptoms of obstructive BPH or an increase in urinary flow. Since not all men demonstrate a response to Proscar, those who have large amounts of residual urine or who have severe obstructive symptoms are not candidates for treatment with this drug, particularly since the treatment has to be continued for at least six months before any improvement can be appreciated. Patients should be evaluated by urinary flow rate and bladder sonogram for determination of residual urine and PSA levels prior to initiation of treatment, and these studies should be repeated in six months after the treatment has started to determine the effect of the drug.

IV. TREATMENTS UNDER INVESTIGATION

A. Hormonal Manipulation. The first attempt at treatment of clinical BPH with hormone manipulation was reported as early as 1895 in an experiment involving 111 men with obstructive BPH who underwent castration. Of those surviving the operation, 87 percent showed rapid decrease of prostate volume.

Since that time, innumerable experiments to treat obstructive BPH have been conducted using hormone manipulation in which shrinkage of the prostate has been demonstrated, generally by 30 percent. These studies have demonstrated the endocrine relationship between the male hormones and prostate enlargement, but this form of treatment has little appeal because of the inevitable loss of libido, and often subsequent impotence.

Other methods of blocking the action of androgens (male hormones) have attracted interest for many years. Medications such as Cyproterone, Flutamide, Medroxiprogesterone and LHRH Agonists have all been studied, but none of them found a useful place in managing patients with symptoms of BPH, mainly because of either loss of sexual function, or associated cost, or side effects.

B. TRANSURETHRAL LASER-INDUCED PROSTATECTOMY (TULIP). Transurethral laser prostatectomy, generally referred to by the acronym TULIP, is a new procedure under investigation for relieving prostate obstruction by delivering laser energy to the prostate. This procedure is different from the Visual Laser Prostatectomy described earlier. Patients who undergo laser prostatectomy do not require hospitalization, since there is no postoperative bleeding. The procedure requires only regional or local anesthesia, and the urethra heals rapidly. During the first two weeks after treatment patients generally complain of irritation while voiding, presumably due to swelling caused by the laser radiation.

The TULIP system consists of a probe containing an optical laser fiber and paired ultrasound transducers. The probe is passed inside a balloon, which when inflated in the prostatic urethra, permits 100 percent transmission of ultrasound and laser energy while holding the prostate tissue in place (Fig. 4-2). In addition to compressing the tissue

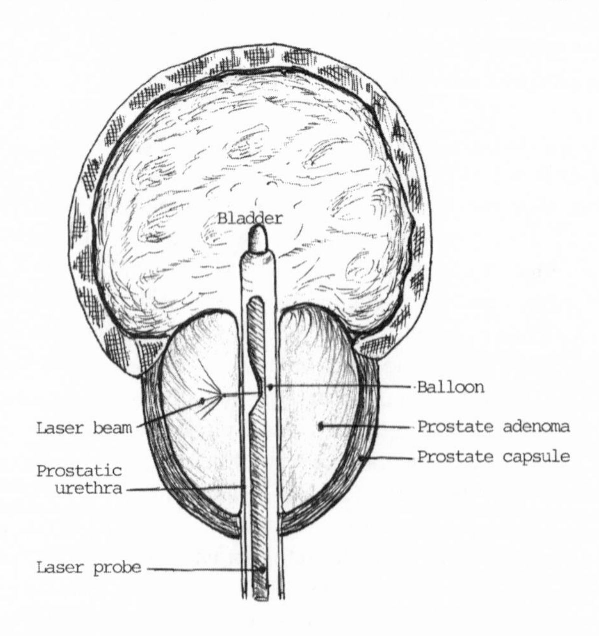

Figure 4-2. Transurethral laser-induced prostatectomy.

and making it more uniform, the inflatable balloon decreases the blood supply, therefore permitting better laser penetration.

On the basis of experimentation with the first thirty patients who have been treated under the FDA-approved protocol, it appears that TULIP provides accurate destruction of obstructive prostate tissue. It seems to show promise as a safe and effective alternative to TURP. TULIP is still under investigation and is not FDA-approved for general use as of this writing.

C. Hyperthermia (Microwaving of Prostate). Microwaving prostate obstruction (hyperthermia) is the delivery of a desired and controlled form of heat to a diseased organ while protecting the surrounding healthy tissue from irreversible damage. Early treatments using hyperthermia were directed at cancer. Diseased tissue is treated at 40 to 42 degrees centigrade, temperatures at which malignant tissue is more susceptible to permanent damage than benign tissue. At temperatures below 40 degrees centigrade, neither malignant nor normal cells seem to show much effect; at temperatures above 45 degrees centigrade, both malignant and normal cells are affected by heat, and cell death occurs.

Extensive testing in Europe has not revealed any significant complications associated with the use of hyperthermia. Since this form of treatment does not preclude later TURP, many patients may prefer this simple, safe, outpatient procedure that does not affect potency and permits return to normal activities much sooner than when TURP is performed. Reports from England, Belgium and France indicate that 70 to 75 percent of patients treated with hyperthermia have significant improvement in symptoms of prostate obstruction, with improvement in peak flow rates and reduction in the amount of residual urine. Most patients so treated go back to their normal activities the next day, and only a few have required postoperative catheterization. The procedure is done on an outpatient basis, and can in some cases be performed under local anesthesia with intravenous sedation.

As of this writing, hyperthermia in the United States is experimental, but within the next two years it may become available as an alternative to TURP. There are a number of issues to be resolved in the coming years that will determine the role this treatment will play in the management of patients with BPH.

Tissue treated with heat results in scarring of the prostatic tissue in the immediate vicinity of the urethra. These changes in turn result in the shrinkage of the periurethral prostate, diminishing the static component of prostate enlargement.

During the summer of 1990, a French company, Technomed International, released a new device called the Prostatron. The Prostatron uses microwaves and has been used extensively in many European medical institutions to treat BPH. But in the United States, the FDA only recently gave Technomed approval to begin Prostatron clinical trials at five American institutions over the next two years. A water-cooled urethral balloon catheter (Fig. 4-3) houses a metal antenna that delivers heat through an aperture close to the balloon. After the catheter is inserted into the bladder, the balloon is inflated and drawn by traction into the bladder neck, placing the antenna outlet immediately below the prostate. A rectal thermometer is inserted into the rectum immediately adjacent to the gland to measure temperature. After preliminary urethral cooling, the microwave antenna raises prostatic temperature to 45 to 50 degrees centigrade, causing the rectal thermometer to register 42 to 43 degrees centigrade. These temperatures are maintained for one hour. As a safety mechanism, rectal readings above these levels automatically interrupt power supply.

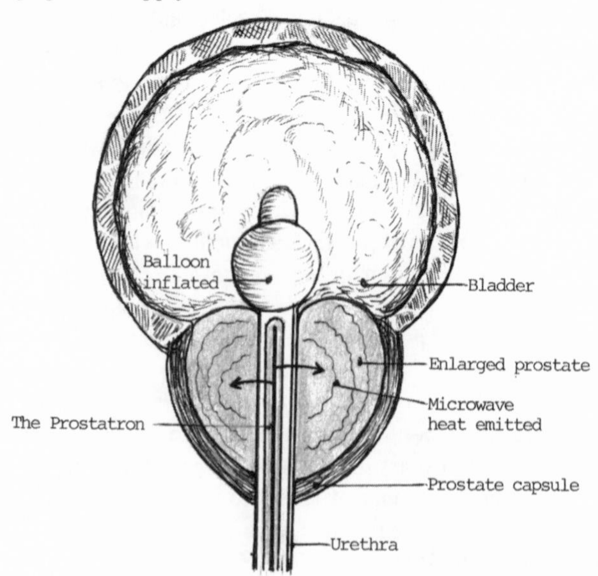

Figure 4-3. The Prostatron: designed to microwave prostate obstruction.

Transurethral microwave hyperthermia appears to be a safe, effective, and conservative treatment for patients with BPH who would otherwise require standard surgical treatment.

D. Prostate Stents

Metallic Stents. In the constant search for alternatives to conventional surgical treatment for BPH, intraprostatic stents have been developed. These would be used only in patients who are unfit for surgery because their medical problems are of such magnitude that surgery and anesthesia pose a significant risk. Until long-term results are reported, the stents cannot be recommended in patients who otherwise are candidates for surgery. There are two types of metallic stents: microporous tubular meshes and metallic spirals.

Microporous Tubular Meshes. These were originally developed for use in blood vessels, then were used for urethral strictures, and more recently have been inserted into the prostatic urethra. The prosthesis is made of metal woven into a self-expandable tubular mesh (Fig. 4-4). When placed in the prostatic urethra the mesh expands to become a flexible but stable cylinder, large enough to allow the passage of a catheter should it become necessary. By virtue of the mesh's pores, urothelium (lining of the bladder and urethra) grows through to cover the stent following placement. This feature differentiates the microporous stents from other stents. In men, the lining of the urethra has been seen to cover the stent within three months. Microporous stents should be considered permanent once epithelialization (covering by

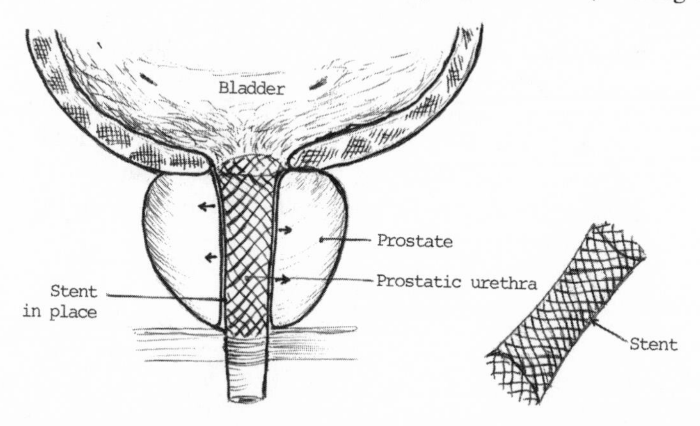

Figure 4-4. A tubular-mesh metallic stent placed in the prostatic urethra. The stent compresses the obstructive BPH and opens the prostatic urethra.

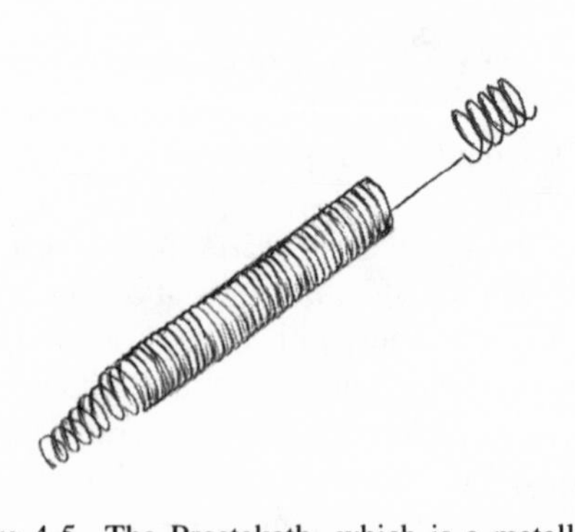

Figure 4-5. The Prostakath, which is a metallic spiral.

urethral lining) is complete. At present these stents have tended to be restricted to patients who, owing to current medical illnesses, are either unfit for surgery or have a limited life expectancy. Because of the lack of long-term follow-up, their use in younger, fitter patients cannot be recommended.

Metallic Spirals. The spirals consist of a tightly coiled metallic spring that lodges in the prostatic urethra. In contrast to the microporous mesh, the device does not become covered with epithelium and thus remains a foreign body in the urethra for as long as it remains in place.

Placement of these stents can be done under local anesthesia, and no significant complications have been reported. Symptoms of urgency, frequency of urination, and irritative symptoms disappear within three months.

Preliminary data from the United States and England appear to show that the use of stents to relieve bladder outlet obstruction from an enlarged prostate is reasonable and effective. These devices have not been approved by the FDA and they are not, therefore, available for widespread clinical use. However, stents are under clinical investigation in FDA-monitored clinical trials, and it is expected that they will soon be available for general use.

CHAPTER 5

Cancer of the Prostate

Incidence and Causation

Cancer is a general term used for a group of conditions distinguished by uncontrolled cell growth. Each type of cancer has its own name, growth pattern, treatment, and chances of control or cure.

The human body is made up of billions of cells. Normally, cells wear out, die, and are replaced in a very orderly and carefully controlled manner. This results in an appropriate number of cells, organized to form tissues and organs that perform specific functions. Sometimes, however, cells are replaced in a way that is out of control, that lacks the organization and order needed for normal function. The abnormal, uncontrolled, and disorderly growth of cells form an accumulation of cells called a malignant tumor, cancerous tumor, or simply cancer.

The cancer cells exploit their new freedom. They obey no laws, follow no rules, do not stay in place, and do not perform any function for the benefit of the whole organism. They reproduce without control. Cancer cells can develop the tendency to multiply, invade other organs, and destroy them, or they can enter body fluids, such as blood and lymph, and thus allow malignant cells to spread to other parts of the body. This process is called **metastasis**.

While everyone is familiar with blood, most people know very little about lymph. Lymph is a clear fluid that drains waste from cells. This fluid travels through vessels called lymphatic channels and drains into small bean-shaped structures called lymph nodes. These nodes filter undesirable substances such as bacteria and tumor cells (Fig. 5-1).

When a patient is confronted with the diagnosis of prostate cancer,

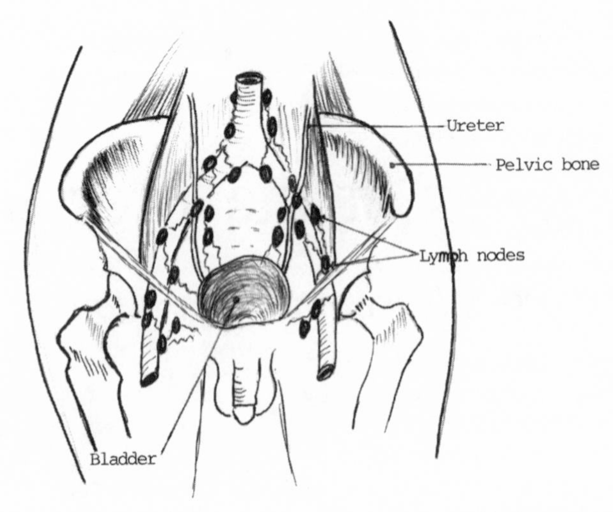

Figure 5-1. The distribution of the pelvic lymph nodes, which filter tumor cells.

one of his immediate concerns is whether it can be cured or not. What are his chances of cure? Will he die soon? Is it too late for cure, or will he go on to live a productive life? When cancer of the prostate is diagnosed early, before it has spread outside the capsule, chances of cure are excellent. The rate of tumor growth can vary widely from patient to patient. Some men can live for many years even after cancer has spread to his bones if the patient responds to appropriate treatment.

Incidence of Prostate Cancer

The risk of developing cancer of the prostate increases with age. Cancer of the prostate is primarily a disease of older men; it occurs most often in men over fifty-five years of age, and more than 80 percent of cases are diagnosed in men over the age of sixty-five. The American Cancer Society estimates that one of every 10 men will develop prostate cancer by age 85.

Prostate cancer is the most frequent cancer affecting men. It is estimated that this year (1993) prostate cancer will develop in 165,000 men and 35,000 will die of it, in the United States alone. A male newborn has a 10 percent chance of developing prostate cancer and about a 3.5 percent chance of dying of it during his lifetime. The reported mortality rate of prostate cancer has increased steadily over the past thirty years; it now ranks behind lung cancer as the second leading cause of cancer death among American men.

Its occurrence is increasing as the mean age of the population increases, and the high mortality is due in part to the low percentage of patients who are diagnosed in the disease's early stages, when the tumor is still localized in the prostate. By the time the diagnosis of prostate cancer is made, frequently the cancer has spread already and is therefore not curable. Current available treatments rarely cure, unless the tumor is still localized.

The discrepancy between the incidence of prostate cancer and its death rate is a clear suggestion that prostate cancer in many cases is of a very low-grade malignancy, that it grows very slowly, and that men often die *with* the disease rather than *from* it. It is generally recognized that regardless of the modality of treatment, patients who have low-grade (well-differentiated), early-stage tumors will do very well, while patients who have high-grade (poorly differentiated) tumors have a poor prognosis. During the past few years, researchers have become aware that tumor volume has also a great prognostic value. Among these researchers, Dr. T. A. Stamey and Dr. J. E. McNeil of Stanford University have clearly shown that the larger the tumor volume at the time the diagnosis is made, the greater the chance that the tumor will be of a higher grade, and therefore carry a poorer prognosis. It thus appear that microscopic grade and volume are the strongest predictors of survival.

Causes of Prostate Cancer

The cause of prostate cancer is not known; however, based on epidemiologic observations, several factors have been suggested as being predisposing factors to prostate cancer.

Genetic Factors

It is difficult to separate genetic from environmental factors. Several studies over the years have reported a higher incidence of prostate cancer among relatives of prostate cancer patients; however, studies of specific genetic typing have not confirmed this occurrence. There are significant national and racial differences in the incidence of and mortality from prostate cancer. For instance, northern European and North American countries have relatively high rates; Latin American and southern European countries have intermediate rates; and eastern European and Far Eastern countries have relatively low rates. Some of these differences may be attributable to differences in the detection and reporting of cases.

African-American men have two times more cancer of the prostate than European-Americans. African-American males have the highest incidence of prostate cancer in the world. It is reported that they develop prostate cancer at an earlier age than whites and tend to present with a higher stage of disease. In contrast, Native Americans, Hispanics, and Orientals have a significantly lower incidence than whites. The differences between countries in mortality rate and clinical prostate cancer are striking. The United States is near the high end of the spectrum, whereas Japan is near the low end.

Interestingly, Japanese immigrants in the United States and their descendants show increase in clinical incidence and mortality that are close to United States rates. These findings strongly suggest that there are unidentified environmental promoting factors.

Hormonal Factors

Several observations have suggested that certain hormonal factors may be important in the development of prostate cancer. These include:

- Most prostate cancers seem ''dependent'' on male hormones (androgens)
- Prostate cancer does not often develop in men who have lost both testes

Environmental Factors

Several environmental factors have been proposed as playing a possible role in development of prostate cancer. These include:

- Exposure to automobile exhaust fumes
- Air pollution
- Cadmium fertilizers
- Certain chemicals in the rubber, printing, painting, and shipfitting industries

The validity of these associations is open to question, and no evidence has been found that these factors cause cancer of the prostate. Cigarette smoke does not seem to have any significant impact either.

Infectious Agents

A variety of infectious agents have been considered as possible cause of prostate cancer, including cytomegalovirus, RNA virus, and herpes virus. As yet, no study has demonstrated that these agents cause cancer of the prostate.

In many ways, prostate cancer is very similar to breast cancer in women. Both diseases are lethal. The American Cancer Society estimates that breast cancer will kill 46,000 women and 300 men in the United States in 1993; prostate cancer will kill 35,000 men in 1993. Breast cancer strikes a little earlier in life than prostate cancer. The median age of women who develop breast cancer is about sixty years, whereas seventy-two is the median age for men when cancer of the prostate strikes. Both diseases can be treated and cured if detected early enough.

Although the two cancers are relatively comparable, the attention paid to them is not. While cancer of the breast has received significant attention from the research community, far less funding has been dedicated to prostate cancer research, and far fewer routine examinations are done in men.

This disparity in attention would seem easily explainable. For one thing, breasts have cosmetic importance, they are visible, and both men and women have become fascinated by them, while the prostate is tucked deep in the pelvis, where it can't be seen. Screening for prostate cancer is far less pleasant than a mammogram examination of the breast. Many men still have difficulty allowing the physician to probe into a very private part of their anatomy.

Public relations in favor of early detection of breast cancer has been active for quite some time, and an annual mammogram, particularly after age forty-five, is recommended by many doctors. In contrast, many men barely know they have a prostate, let alone what can go wrong with it. For quite some time, many celebrities have been open about their cancer of the breast, yet it has not been until very recently that cancer of the prostate has received attention, thanks to the efforts of courageous national celebrities like Senators Alan Cranston, Robert Dole and Ted Stevens. These men and others have spoken out publicly about their disease and taken the common prostate cancer out of the closet.

Recently, Senator Robert Dole has spoken out on testing and treatment for prostate cancer. After he had surgery to treat his prostate cancer, he appeared on national television programs to discuss the disease, and his office has been bombarded by hundreds of phone calls and letters from men newly diagnosed with the same cancer who said they had gone for testing only after hearing the senator speak of his experience. If other public figures follow the leadership of Senator Dole, we will soon have enough funding and public support to step up research and to learn about this killer.

This common disease, which has largely gone unmentioned by those whose lives have been stunned by it, may be entering a new era in its history, as more and more men, encouraged by those in the public eye, seek an examination from their physicians and have their disease detected at a stage where it is still curable.

CHAPTER 6

Cancer of the Prostate

Symptoms, Diagnosis, and Screening

Symptoms of Prostate Cancer

Early in the course of the disease, prostate cancer may produce no symptoms. The only clinical evidence of cancer may be induration, or hardening, of the prostate discovered during digital rectal examination. Induration in some patients may not be detectable. In some cases a discrete nodule may be present in the prostate.

A significant number of men with prostate cancer also have benign prostate enlargement; in these cases the symptoms may be due to obstruction, and it may have been the obstructive symptoms that made these patients seek medical attention. Frequently, patients who have prostate cancer have no detectable induration or hard nodules but their cancer is discovered on microscopic examination of the prostate adenoma removed because of benign obstructive enlargement. In these cases the cancer is found unexpectedly, and if it has not spread, it can be cured.

In advanced disease, when the malignancy has spread to bones, patients may experience severe bone pain, most frequently in the lower back, hips, and upper parts of the thighs. If the cancer has spread to the spine, it may cause compression of the spinal cord. In these cases a variety of symptoms may develop, such as numbness of the legs, muscular weakness, difficulty in walking, and, in severe cases, inability to walk or move the legs. Difficulty in walking or the inability to walk due to paralysis constitute real emergencies and patients with these problems must have immediate therapy to decompress the spinal cord.

The neurosurgeon in these cases removes a small part of the vertebral bone that is causing pressure on the spinal cord. The operation is generally successful, and sometimes the improvement is dramatic. A drug, ketoconazole, which has antiandrogen action also gives immediate relief and is the recommended nonsurgical treatment.

In some advanced cases the tumor may spread to the base of the bladder and obstruct the channels that carry the urine from the kidneys into the bladder (ureters). If both ureters are obstructed the kidneys cannot drain urine properly and uremic poisoning develops. This situation may require decompression of the obstructed kidneys, such as by inserting a tube directly into one or both kidneys.

In extreme cases—when the patient is very old, is not expected to live long, and is not having pain from the obstruction—the family and the doctor may decide to not give any further treatment and to let the patient die peacefully and painlessly from uremia.

Screening Prostate Cancer

As the population ages, the incidence of prostate cancer is expected to increase significantly, creating a greater need for better methods of early detection, staging, and treatment. Because of our inability to prevent prostate cancer, early detection offers the most practical method of reducing mortality. The American Cancer Society and the American Urological Association recommend annual prostate specific antigen (PSA) level blood testing and rectal examination beginning at age fifty years for the early detection of prostate cancer, and beginning at age forty years for the high-risk men such as those with a strong family history of prostate cancer, and for African-American men. In the February 17, 1993, issue of the *Journal of the American Medical Association (JAMA)* an article was published on the results of two well-designed studies reporting a possible link between vasectomy and prostate cancer. The National Institute of health and the American Urological Association took this report seriously, and formed a blue ribbon panel on vasectomy and prostate cancer. The panel, after significant research and studies, found no causal relationship between vasectomy and increased insidence of prostate cancer. In addition, preliminary data analysis involving more than 35,000 men screened during the 1992 Prostate Cancer Awareness Week showed no such association. The panel reported the results of the studies during the American Urological

Association's 88th annual meeting in June of 1993 and recommended no special screening for men who have had a vasectomy.

Unfortunately, few men voluntarily request the procedure, and physicians often neglect this simple preventative measure. A prostate nodule or an area of induration is an important finding; microscopic examination reveals cancerous cells in approximately 50 percent of all nodules discovered during rectal examination. In about 40 percent of these malignant prostate nodules, tumor cells have spread outside the prostate by the time they are discovered.

Early detection clearly improves a patient's chances for cure, and even if the cancer cannot be eradicated, earlier detection, combined with current available therapies, can markedly improve the patient's quality of life. Other screening methods are being investigated, but at present DRE remains the most popular and cost-effective approach for early detection of prostate cancer in a large population.

To effectively recommend widespread screening, we first need to improve disease awareness, particularly among older men. A recent screening campaign and survey conducted by the Prostate Cancer Education Council revealed that almost two-thirds of the 10,000 men surveyed had not had a physical examination within the past year, and that of those who did, less than half had had a rectal examination! The council also reported that 14 percent of those surveyed had never had a rectal examination, and that only 18 percent had had one within the past twelve months. Educational campaigns and screenings have met with mixed results. Part of the problem, no doubt, is the nature of the rectal examination. Many men are still reluctant to have periodic rectal examinations, considering it an invasion of their privacy. Although DRE is quick, painless, and requires no preparation, most men must overcome a psychological barrier against allowing a stranger to probe inside their rectum.

Digital Rectal Examination

DRE has been described in the first chapter of this book, but its importance cannot be overemphasized. Wearing a rubber glove, the examiner places the well-lubricated forefinger on the anal opening and gently presses until the sphincter relaxes. The finger is slowly inserted through the anal canal, with the pad of the finger kept facing the anterior wall of the rectum. The examiner will feel the prostate as an elastic, bulging surface that has the consistency of the tip of the nose. The examiner will feel the size and consistency and will check for hard or firm nodules and for areas of induration. Cancer of the prostate classically presents with a hard area or nodule palpable on digital exam. However, cancer may be present even when the gland feels normal, since the entire gland cannot be felt on rectal examination and the areas of cancer may be small.

Prostate Specific Antigen (PSA)

PSA is a protein that was first isolated in 1970. It is only found in prostate cells, is produced by both benign and malignant prostate tissue. It has the tendency to become elevated in the majority of men with prostate cancer. PSA testing is very simple. A blood sample is obtained and sent to a reputable laboratory. The normal levels of PSA in blood are 0-2.5 ng/ml using the Yang technique and 0-4 ng/ml using the Hybritech technique.

Unfortunately, elevations occur in BPH as well as in cancer, making the marker prostate-specific but not cancer-specific, and therefore ineffective as an initial screening tool. PSA has a number of applications in the management of patients with known prostate cancer, and can be used in staging established disease. But perhaps the greatest use of PSA determination is in the monitoring of patients after surgical removal of the prostate. Since prostate tissue is the only source of PSA, there should be no detectable PSA after curative removal of the prostate. In the absence of prostate cells, PSA should be close to zero. Detectable levels of this protein after radical prostatectomy for cure of prostate cancer indicates that not all prostate cells have been removed, and this means that the patient has either recurrence or residual tumor. Patients with detectable levels of PSA after surgery may have microscopic undetected malignant cells in the pelvic lymph nodes, at the surgical margins, or elsewhere in the body.

In addition, PSA is an excellent predictor for response to androgen deprivation therapy (therapy directed to eliminate male hormones), often falling dramatically after the institution of such therapy.

Over the past number of years, PSA has received a great deal of publicity through the news media. Unfortunately, this publicity, although well intentioned, has been misleading, and some men believe that the test will determine whether or not they have cancer. During the past year, in our practice in Alexandria, Virginia, we have had patients come to our office for PSA testing to see if they have cancer. There is understandable disappointment when they discover about the real purpose of the test.

Prostate Acid Phosphatase (PAP)

PAP is also a protein secreted by the prostate after puberty. It has the tendency to rise above normal levels when cancer of the prostate has extended beyond the prostate capsule. While an increase in the blood levels of this enzyme may indicate advanced prostate cancer, it can also be elevated in benign prostate hypertrophy (BPH). The disadvantages of this protein in contrast to PSA is that it is not specific to the prostate (there are other organs that produce it) and it can be elevated in conditions other than prostate disease. For this reason, many urologists have virtually abandoned the use of PAP in favor of PSA. It may, however, have a role in staging of prostate cancer, since it tends to be elevated only when the tumor has spread beyond the confines of the prostate.

Diagnosing Prostate Cancer

A significant number of patients suffering from prostate cancer may not have symptoms at all, and diagnosis is often dependent on suspicion raised during routine physical examination. Although rectal examination may be suggestive of prostate carcinoma, diagnosis is made by microscopic (pathologic) examination of prostate tissue.

Biopsy of the prostate

Biopsy of the prostate is the removal of a small fragment of the prostate tissue for examination under the microscope. This can be done in several ways, but the most common is needle biopsy. There are two different methods of performing needle biopsy of the prostate gland: core needle biopsy and fine needle aspiration biopsy.

Core Needle Biopsy

This is a good and reliable method of diagnosing prostate cancer. A specially designed hollow needle is used to remove a small fragment of prostate tissue. Traditionally, the prostate has been approached with the needle either through the rectum or through the perineum (the area between the scrotum and the anus). During the past few years, transrectal ultrasound (TRUS) of the prostate became available, and with it the ability to perform ultrasound guided needle biopsy. This procedure has been so successful that the perineal approach has become obsolete.

Ultrasound is used to guide a biopsy needle directly into the suspicious area in the prostate. Using the automotive spring-loaded biopsy gun and a biopsy needle, the urologist can take multiple small cores of tissue from precisely identified areas of the prostate (Figs. 6-1, 6-2 and also Fig. 2-8). The procedure can be easily accomplished in the physician's office, anesthesia is not required.

After the ultrasound probe is passed into the rectum, an image of the prostate appears on a TV screen and a marker line indicates the path the needle will take when fired. The needle is then fired. Broad spectrum antibiotics are used beginning the day before the procedure and continued for the next 24 to 48 hours afterward.

The Controversy Over Screening for Prostate Cancer

Screening programs for prostate cancer encourage early detection of the disease, and are geared toward decreasing mortality from cancer of the prostate.

Today, existing screening programs consist of determination of PSA levels in blood and digital rectal examination. There have been several recent reports that up to 30 percent of patients with early prostate cancer have normal PSA levels. Furthermore, since many men with benign prostate hypertrophy will have elevated levels of PSA, using these tests for screening may result in many unnecessary biopsies. On the other hand, several studies have concluded that digital rectal examination of the prostate fails to detect a significant number of men with early cancer.

A study sponsored by the Prostate Cancer Education Council compared the results of PSA and DRE screenings during the 1989 Prostate Awareness Week. More than 14,000 men were screened in hospitals and clinics across the United States. Data from five centers were collected on patients who had DRE and PSA results, and reports were presented at a recent meeting of the American Urological Association. The cancer detection rate for DRE was 2.6 percent, compared with 5 percent for PSA. The most important point of the data is that 35 percent

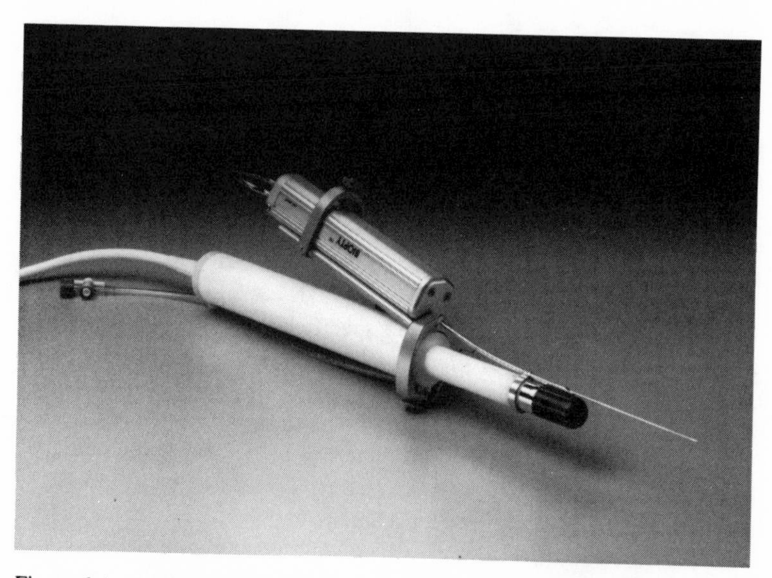

Figure 6-1. An ultrasound probe used in transrectal ultrasound of the prostate. A spring mechanism gun is attached to the probe, which, when fired, allows the examiner to obtain a needle biopsy of the prostate. (*Courtesy Teknar, Inc.*)

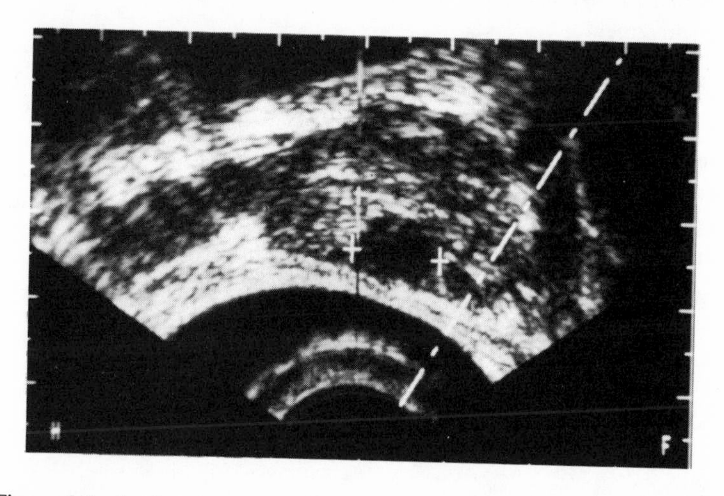

Figure 6-2. An image of the prostate gland as it appears on the television screen. Prostate cancer appears as a darker area between the two white crosses. (*Courtesy Teknar, Inc.*)

of the cancers found were in patients who had normal glands on DRE but elevated PSA. A similar report was recently published from a prostate cancer screening program conducted by the Department of Urology at Stanford University. Each of 478 men had DRE and PSA screenings. The study concluded that PSA was a more powerful screening tool for prostate cancer than DRE.

An ideal screening test would be one that is positive only when prostate cancer is present. The test or tests used in screening would have to be very sensitive and specific enough to detect early cancer. In other words, both the sensitivity and the specificity would have to be 100 percent. Today, as the sensitivity declines, more patients with prostate cancer go undetected; as the specificity decreases, more patients undergo unnecessary biopsies. The ideal test is not yet available.

Critics of screening for prostate cancer point out that only a fraction of prostate cancer patients will die of their disease, that many patients die *with* the disease rather than *from* it, and that it is therefore not desirable to diagnose and treat all men with prostate cancer, especially now that TRUS can detect tumors less than 1 cm in diameter. Because there is no method for distinguishing small cancerous tumors that will remain dormant from those that will metastasize and kill, there is a potential for overdetection and overtreatment of patients who may not need treatment.

These facts need to be taken into account but we must not forget that the expected mortality from prostate cancer in the United States is approximately 35,000 men this year (1993). This staggering figure is a reflection of the fact that much more research is needed to identify which cancerous tumors are likely to progress and which will remain dormant. If that were known, treatment could be selected only for those patients who are at risk of dying of their disease. Until then, screening for prostate cancer will remain a controversial issue.

CHAPTER 7

Grading and Staging of Prostate Cancer

Grading and Staging of Prostate Cancer

Not all cases of cancer of the prostate have the same malignancy potential. Many men over the age of sixty-five have microscopic foci of cancer in their prostates, but the majority of these men die with the disease rather than from it. Some men suffering from prostate cancer can live for many years after the diagnosis is made without ever having symptoms or difficulty from the disease. On the other hand, some men have died of metastases a year or two after being diagnosed. It is the microscopic (pathologic) grade and volume of the cancer that appears to be the strongest predictor of survival in cancer of the prostate. Patients with low-grade malignancy do well, while those with high-grade malignancy or more than 3 cc in cancer volume tend to respond poorly to treatment.

Once cancer of the prostate is diagnosed, it is important to determine what stage it has reached. There are many methods of staging, but in the United States, the most common method has been the Whitmore-Jewitt system which divides the disease into four stages A, B, C, and D, and appears to be the simplest (Fig. 7-1).

Stage A Cancer is a cancer that is not felt on digital rectal examination. It is diagnosed by microscopic examination of prostate tissue removed at the time of surgery performed for what was thought to be benign prostate enlargement.

About 10 percent of patients who undergo prostatectomy for presumed benign disease are found to have cancer. Stage A tumors are confined to the prostate gland. Stage A disease is further divided into A_1 and A_2 categories. In A_1 disease, the tumor covers only a small area of less than 5 percent of the total tissue removed and is a low-removed grade malignancy. If the tumor is bigger than this, or appears to be a high-grade malignancy, the cancer is considered to be an A_2 lesion.

Stage B Cancer exists if the tumor is palpable on rectal examination as a hard nodule. This stage is also subdivided, into B_1 and B_2, depending on whether the palpable tumor or nodule is small (2 cm or less in diameter) or large (more than 2 cm in diameter). Perhaps 20 to 30 percent of men with prostate cancer have Stage B disease when it is initially diagnosed. It is to diagnose this stage of tumor that annual digital rectal examination of the prostate is recommended. As in the case of Stage A prostate cancer, Stage B lesions are also confined to the prostate and are curable.

Stage C Cancer is more advanced and larger than the A or B stage. It has spread to the seminal vesicles or extended through the prostate capsule. On digital rectal examination the entire prostate feels hard, and sometimes feels as if it has extended up behind the base of the prostate and into the seminal vesicles. About 30 to 40 percent of all prostate cancers are in this stage when first diagnosed. As in Stages A and B, Stage C does not produce any symptoms and the patient is not aware of having the life-threatening condition.

Stage D Cancer is a cancer that has spread beyond the confines of the prostate, has produced distant metastasis, or has spread to the pelvic lymph nodes. As in Stages A and B, Stage D is also subdivided, into D_1 and D_2. In Stage D_1 the tumor has spread only into regional lymph nodes of the pelvis. If the cancer has produced distance metastasis to other organs such as the lungs or bones, it is considered a Stage D_2 lesion. Bone metastasis usually produces pain, which can be very severe. Stage D disease cannot be cured, but it can be controlled.

Grading of the tumor is also very important. Grading refers to the degree of malignancy, or the degree of cellular change from the normal. In medical terms, this change or transformation is called differentiation. Well-differentiated tumors resemble normal cells and have low malignancy potential, while poorly differentiated tumors have little or no resemblance to normal cells. The more poorly differentiated the tumor the more malignant its behavior.

The most commonly used method of grading in the United States is the Gleason system. It is done by the pathologist, who assigns what is

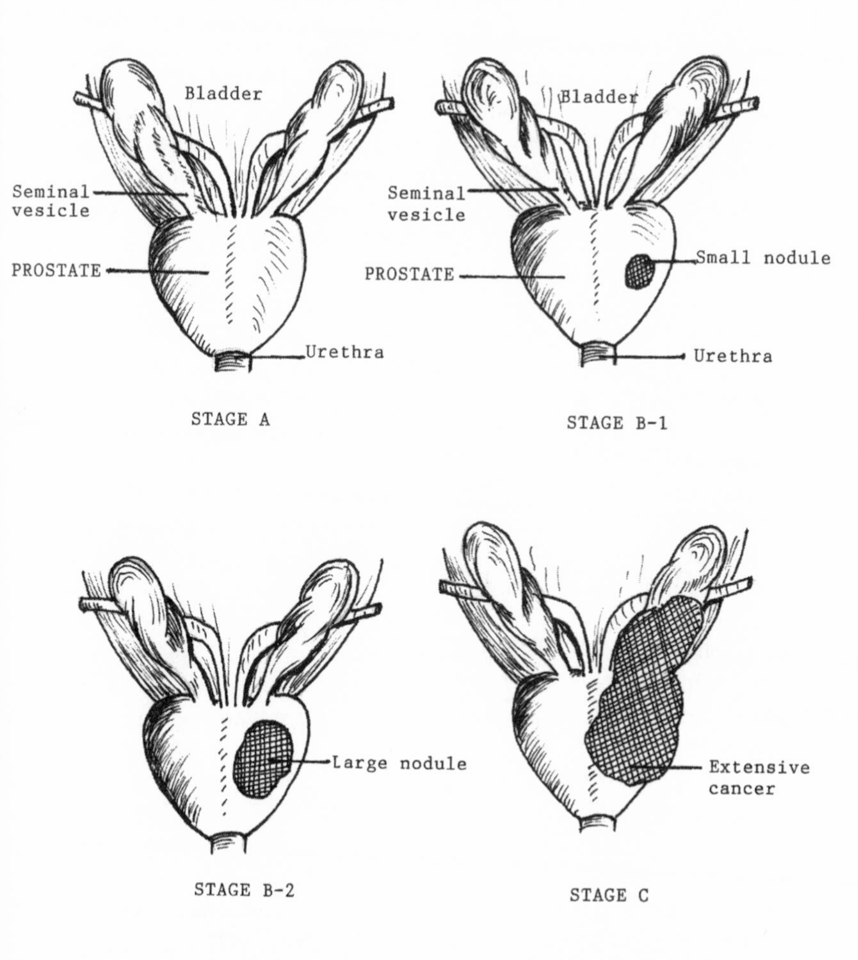

Figure 7-1. The prostate gland showing the different stages of cancer.

Stage A. This is the "occult" stage of prostate cancer, in which the cancer is not palpable on rectal examination.
Stage B-1. Cancer is palpable on digital examination as a small nodule measuring 2 cm or less.
Stage B-2. In this stage the cancer is palpable as a larger module of more than 2 cm.
Stage C. The cancer is extensive and has invaded the seminal vesicles and the prostate capsule.
Stage D (not shown). In this stage the cancer has metastasized to pelvic lymph nodes or other organs.

called a "Gleason Score" from 1 to 10 to the tissue. Another technique for grading is the "flow cytometry," which examines the DNA composition of individual cells and grades them according to their degree of malignancy potential. This method is very promising, but much more research is needed for it to become highly useful in grading prostate cancer.

Staging Procedures

Once a biopsy has reported a malignancy, the physician wants to know whether the tumor is confined to the gland and is curable, or whether it has spread locally or to other organs. There are several tests that he or she may like to perform to know just how extensive the cancer is. This study is called staging, because the doctor is trying to find out the stage of the disease. The ideal study is not yet available, but several tests are helpful. The following are the most useful tests performed for this purpose:

- Bone Scan
- Computerized Axial Tomography (CAT scan)
- Magnetic Resonance Imaging (MRI)
- Pelvic Lymphadenectomy (lymph node dissection or removal of lymph nodes), which can be performed either through open surgery or by means of laparoscopy

Bone Scan

This is a simple and very informative test, and it is the one usually done as soon as the diagnosis of cancer of the prostate is made. It will tell the doctor if the bones are involved with the tumor (metastasis). Bone scans are much more sensitive in diagnosing metastasis than conventional X-ray studies. One of the most common places to which prostate cancer spreads is the bones, particularly those of the spine, hips, pelvis, and the upper part of the leg bones. A small amount of a radioisotope material is injected intravenously, which then goes to all bones in the body within two hours. Two hours after injection, the patient is placed on a table and a scanner takes a picture of the entire skeleton. If there is tumor or spread of cancer to the bones, the image of the skeleton obtained shows areas of tumor as darker spots than the rest of the bone.

Darker spots, however, are no proof that the cancer has spread to the bone. Any process that can destroy bone, such as an injury, arthritis, or degenerative bone disease, will result in increased uptake (black spots) on the bone scan (Fig. 7-2). In these cases, conventional X rays are done to detect the presence of certain conditions of the bone that may account for the abnormal scan. If the areas of increased uptake correspond to abnormal bone on the X-ray examinations, then metastatic cancer becomes the most likely diagnosis.

Computerized Axial Tomography (CAT Scan)

Also known as a CT scan, this is an excellent diagnostic study that combines the use of X rays with computer technology. A major advantage of this imaging method over conventional X-ray studies is the greater ability of CT scans to detect differences in density between parts of the body, making it very useful in the evaluation of tumors anywhere in the body (Fig 7-3). It is possible in some cases to determine the extent of spread of a prostate cancer by means of CT scans. CT scans are obtained in patients with cancer of the prostate mainly to see if there is gross involvement of pelvic lymph nodes with tumor, in which case the nodes are enlarged and irregular. But the nodal enlargement is not always due to cancer; sometimes benign inflammation of the nodes can occur, and this would give a false positive picture. On the other hand, there are cases where nodes with tumor may not be enlarged, and this would give a false negative reading. For these reasons, a CT scan is not reliable in all cases.

Magnetic Resonance Imaging (MRI)

This is a radiographic technique that gives a fairly accurate picture of the organs of the body. Like the CT scan, it relies on computer assistance. Its main advantage over CT scanning is that the patient is not exposed to any radiation and there is no known hazard; its only drawback is its high cost. MRI is rapidly becoming the most useful tool for evaluating the prostate and demonstrating extension of disease beyond the confines of the gland (Fig 7-4). A major benefit of MRI imaging is its ability to depict the prostate and adjacent organs clearly and in a variety of orientations, particularly when the rectal probe is utilized. The accuracy of MRI imaging in staging prostate cancer when a device

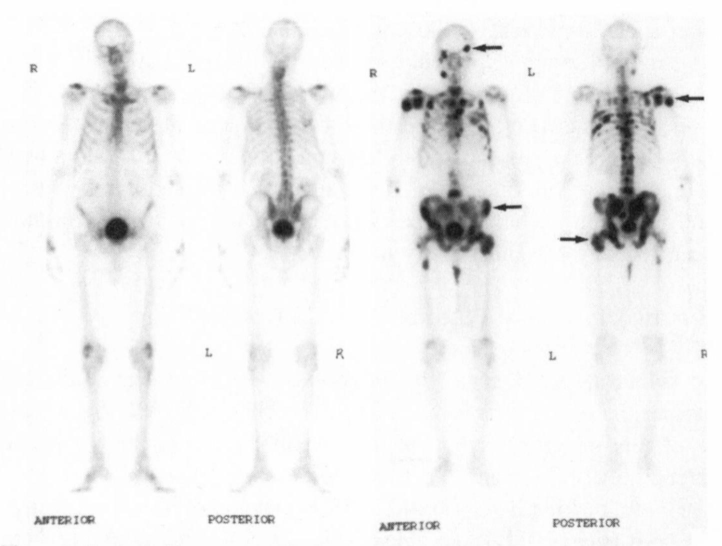

Figure 7-2. Left: Bone scan of a normal man. Right: Bone scan of a man with much metastises, from prostate cancer, shown by arrows.

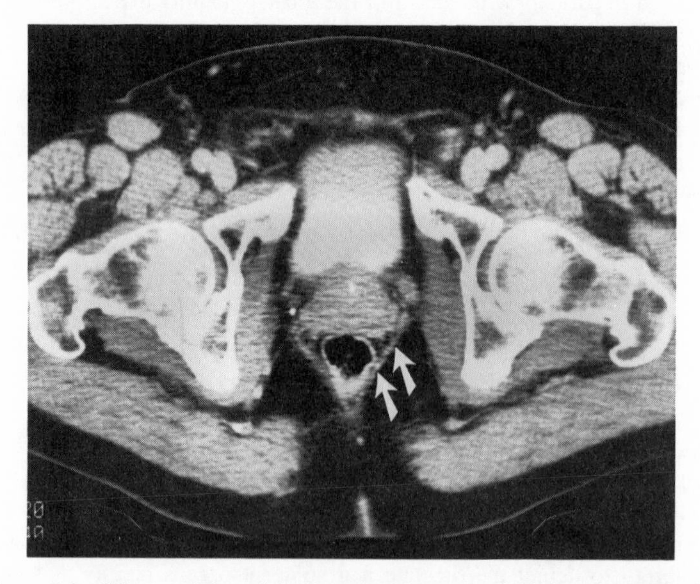

Figure 7-3. CT scan of the pelvis. A major advantage of this imaging method is its ability to defect differences in density between parts of the body. The upper arrow is pointing at the prostate, and the lower at the rectum.

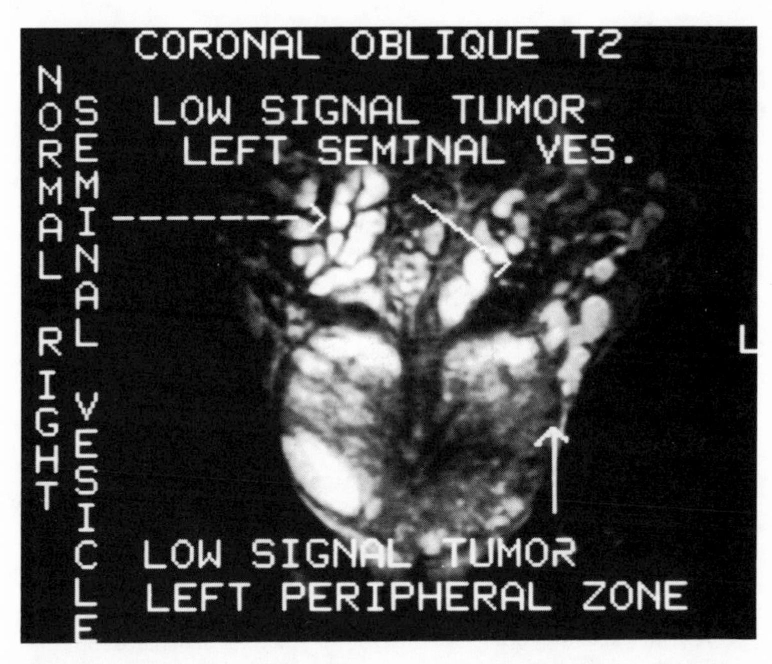

Figure 7-4. An MRI of the prostate and seminal vesicles done through an endorectal coil. It shows the prostate, the seminal vesicles, and cancer of the prostate invading the left seminal vesicle.

called the endorectal coil is used has approached 85 percent in some reports.

Open Lymphadenectomy (Pelvic Lymph Node Dissection)

Conventional lymphadenectomy or lymph node dissection is usually performed through the same incision made for radical prostatectomy. Routinely, the pelvic lymph nodes are removed for microscopic examination just prior to removal of the prostate. Not until the nodes are examined under the microscope and found to be free of malignant invasion can the surgeon be sure that the cancer is confined to the prostate.

Laparoscopic Lymphadenectomy

In laparoscopic lymphadenectomy the urologist uses video technology and highly specialized tools to remove the pelvic lymph nodes, without making a large surgical incision. Instead, the urologist makes four small incisions of less than half an inch each. One of these tiny incisions is made just below the patient's navel so that the surgeon can pass through a special instrument called the laparoscope. The laparoscope is a long, rigid tube that is attached to a miniature video camera and a powerful light. Before the laparoscope is inserted, the patient's abdomen is distended with carbon dioxide gas, which allows the surgeon to see inside the abdomen and pelvis. Once the laparoscope has been inserted, the surgeon guides the laparoscope while watching a TV screen and the view it provides. Three other small incisions are made, one each side and one just above the bladder on the midline. Each of these incisions is used for passage of specialized instruments that remove the lymph nodes. Once the lymph nodes have been cut free, the surgeon removes them though the incision below the navel. After the lymph nodes have been examined under the microscope, the surgeon will decide on the next step. If all nodes removed are negative for cancer, he may then schedule the patient for radiation or for radical prostatectomy.

Although laparoscopic operations have been performed by gynecologists over the past twenty years, general surgeons did not begin performing this technique until about 1988. Since then, laparoscopy has become the method of choice for removing gallbladders. It was not until 1991 that urologists adapted the laparoscopic technique for removal of 2the pelvic lymph nodes, and therefore their experience with the new method is limited. The obvious advantage of the laparoscopic technique is that if the removed nodes are found to have cancer, the patient is spared a major surgical procedure or radiation therapy and other forms of therapy would be indicated.

Advantages of laparoscopic lymph node dissection over the open procedure:

- Very low morbidity
- Rapid return to normal activity

Disadvantages of laparoscopia lymph node dissection:

- Possibility of injury to bowel or blood vessels
- Significant skill and experience are required

CHAPTER 8

Treatment of Prostate Cancer

Treatment of prostate cancer is a very controversial topic. In the United States, current medical thought is that cancer which is limited to the prostate can be cured either by complete removal of the prostate (radical prostatectomy) or by radiation therapy.

One of the factors that has contributed to the controversy over treatment of prostate cancer is that there appears to be some evidence that patients who have cancer localized in the prostate and who have elected not to be treated (opting for what is called "deferred treatment," or simple observation and follow-up) have done just as well as those who underwent either radical prostatectomy or radiation. One of several studies was carried out by the Veterans Administration Cooperative Study. Patients with curable cancer localized in the prostate received either radical prostatectomy plus placebo (sugar pill) or placebo alone. Although the study had significant problems, there was no significant difference in prostate cancer mortality between the two groups.

Treatment of Stage A Cancer

Patients with Stage A cancer are those who had a palpably normal prostate, who then had TURP or prostatectomy for what was thought to be a benign disease, and in whom malignancy was discovered on microscopic examination of prostatic tissue that had been removed from them. Since Stage A cancer is confined to the gland, it can be cured. As mentioned earlier, this stage is diagnosed incidentally and there are no signs or symptoms of cancer. This form of cancer is found in about 10 percent of patients who undergo prostatectomy for obstructive BPH.

Stage A_1 cancer is also called "occult" carcinoma. In this stage the malignancy involves less than 5 percent of the total removed tissue, and is a low-grade, well-differentiated malignancy. The major factors to consider in the treatment of this stage of disease are the age of the patient and his general medical condition. Frequently, these patients are old and suffer from significant cardiovascular or pulmonary problems, and their medical condition limits their life expectancy more than the early prostate cancer would. In this group of patients, definitive treatment is not necessary and simple observation with periodic checkup is all that is required. These patients will most likely die of other causes and have no problem at all with the prostate cancer. Most patients with Stage A_1 (focal) cancer are suitable candidates for this form of observation. Traditionally, these patients have received no other form of treatment.

Recent studies, however, suggest that a significant percentage of these patients are found to have more extensive disease. For this reason, the urologist needs to be sure that the unsuspected, incidental cancer is indeed a Stage A_1 and not merely part of a more extensive disease. Some urologists are recommending a repeat TURP of the prostate in about three months to obtain more tissue for microscopic examination. A selected group of patients with Stage A_1 are currently being treated with radical prostatectomy, but the benefits of such treatment should be carefully weighed against the adverse effects of surgery.

For the patient with a life expectancy of more than fifteen years, Stage A_1 malignancy could eventually be a life-limiting problem. There is some recent evidence that a significant number of patients in this category will eventually develop metastatic disease. Based on these considerations, definitive therapy with radiation, or preferably nerve-sparing radical prostatectomy (removal of the entire prostate), is indicated for these patients.

Of course, not all men fit into these two categories. Between the extremes of the elderly, debilitated man with Stage A_1 cancer who has many medical problems and the healthy sixty-year-old man with the same Stage A_1 cancer who is otherwise in good health, there is a relatively large group of men who do not clearly fit into either group. It is for these patients that urologists recommend a second, more generous TURP of the prostate, if in fact there is more extensive disease.

Patients with Stage A_2 cancer, in sharp contrast with patients who have Stage A_1, have higher-volume tumor, high-grade malignancy, or both. About 25 percent of patients who are clinically considered to have Stage A_2 cancer turn out to have microscopic invasion of the pelvic lymph nodes and therefore have already developed Stage D, or incurable, disease. Cancer progression is much faster, and the death rate much higher, for these patients than for those with A_1 cancer, and aggressive therapy is warranted at the time of diagnosis. Every effort should be made to determine if these patients have any metastases by doing staging tests already described in Chapter 7. However, it is frequently not until the pelvic lymph nodes are removed and examined at the time of radical prostatectomy that one can be sure that these patients in fact have Stage A_2 cancer rather than Stage D disease. Patients with Stage A_2 cancer should be treated with either radiation or, preferably, nerve-sparing radical prostatectomy. These two methods of treatment are described in detail after a brief description of treatment for Stages B, C, and D.

Treatment of Stage B Cancer

In Stage B, a nodule is generally palpable in the prostate (see chapter 7). The cancer is well localized and within the confines of the prostate, and is curable by either radical prostatectomy or by external beam radiation therapy. The efficacy of both treatments is unquestioned, but which treatment offers the best results has been a subject of great controversy.

To resolve issues regarding optimal treatment, the National Cancer Institute and the National Institute of Health convened a Consensus Development Conference on the management of clinically localized prostate cancer in 1987. After presentations and testimony by leading experts in the field, the conclusion of the report stated that for appropriately selected patients, radical prostatectomy and radiation therapy were clearly effective forms of treatment in the attempt to cure cancer limited to the prostate gland; comparisons studies suggested comparable ten-year survival rates with either form of management. What remained unclear was the relative merit of each in producing life-long freedom from cancer recurrence.

The long-term effect of radical prostatectomy had been determined in numerous studies. It did provide cancer-free survival and with a quality of life equivalent to that of a control population free of cancer of comparable age. On the other hand, sufficient long-term follow-up did not yet exist to permit a conclusion about the ability of radiation therapy to eradicate such cancer in an equivalent proportion of patients.

The results of the conference would seem to indicate that radical prostatectomy should be the treatment of choice for patients whose cancer is confined to the prostate.

When the malignancy is truly confined to the prostate and the entire gland is removed, as in the case of a radical prostatectomy, the disease is eradicated and there should be no detectable levels of PSA. In contrast, survival after radiation therapy is frequently with some residual tumor. After radiation of the prostate for cure of prostate cancer, there is always uncertainty as to whether all tumor cells are killed, and when biopsies of the prostate are performed months and even years after radiation, significant numbers of these patients—as many as 60 percent, in some reports—show remaining cancer in their prostate. This is an extremely worrisome occurrence and one of the reasons that many urologists hesitate to recommend radiation for patients who otherwise are suitable candidates for radical prostatectomy.

The meaning of positive biopsies after radiation has been a subject of controversy, but there seems to be increasing evidence in the literature, that these patients with positive biopsies are at high risk of developing metastasis.

For a selected group of patients, as in the case of men with stage A disease, deferred treatment or observation only may be appropriate. This modality of treatment is explained later in this chapter.

Treatment of Stage C Cancer

Stage C cancer of the prostate is more extensive than Stages A and B. The malignancy has generally spread through the capsule or up into the seminal vesicles. Treatment of Stage C disease is even more controversial. There is no agreement on what is the best treatment for Stage C prostate cancer. Various combinations—such as surgery plus hormone therapy, radiation plus hormone therapy, surgery followed by radiation, surgery plus radiation and hormone manipulation, etc.—have been tried, and the results among them are not significantly different in terms of long-term survival, but they are different (better) than *no* treatment.

Stage C cancer is not always established before surgery. Frequently, patients are thought to have Stage B disease and the microscopic examination of the specimen reveals that the cancer has invaded the seminal vesicles, the capsule, or the surgical margins. Rather than initiating hormone manipulation or recommending radiation shortly after surgery, most urologists would probably prefer to follow these patients with periodic levels of PSA; if PSA levels are detectable, then radiation and/or hormone manipulation can be recommended.

Treatment of Stage D Cancer

Stage D prostate cancer is a very serious condition. In Stage D_1 the cancer has spread to pelvic lymph nodes, but has not metastasized to distant organs, and the bone scans are negative. In Stage D_2 there is already distant metastasis to bones, lungs, and other organs. Bone metastasis is readily detectable by means of a bone scan.

Even though in Stage D_1 there is no spread to distant organs, the ability of cancer to proliferate in the pelvic lymph nodes reflects a high probability of metastasis to distant sites, and great malignancy potential. When the pelvic lymph nodes are enlarged and are grossly involved with cancer, this spread can sometimes be detected by MRI or CT scans of the pelvis. In these cases one may suspect Stage D disease. But there are many cases in which the enlarged lymph nodes are not due to a tumor but rather to inflammation. There are other cases where the lymph nodes appear normal in size, yet when removed are found to contain microscopic cancer cells. For these reasons, there is no way of establishing with certainty whether the cancer has spread to one or more of the lymph nodes, short of actual surgical removal of the nodes for examination under the microscope.

Although patients with Stage D_1 disease are not considered to be curable, there are large numbers of patients who have been treated for Stage D_1 with radical prostatectomy or pelvic lymph node dissection in tandem with orchiectomy or hormone manipulation who have been followed for five, ten, and up to fifteen years and are alive and seemingly well. (Patients treated with orchiectomy or hormone manipulation alone have not done as well.) Why these long-term survivals occur in patients with Stage D cancer treated with this combined therapy is not certain, but the only explanation would appear to be that by radical prostatectomy the primary source of cancer is removed, and that it is from the prostate that the metastatic lesions arise. It would make no sense to treat the lymph nodes with radiation and leave the prostate untreated to continue to spill metastatic cells. It is the author's opinion that radiation therapy has no place in the treatment of Stage D_1 cancer, but there are some radiotherapists who disagree. In Stage D_2 cancer that has metastasized to distant organs such as bones or lungs, hormone therapy alone is the treatment of choice.

Hormone Therapy (for Stages C and D)

Hormone therapy, also referred to as "hormone manipulation," is based on the fact that at least 90 percent of prostate cancers are for at least a time dependent upon the male hormone (testosterone) for growth. What this means is that the growth and spread of prostate cancer in at least 90 percent of patients is enhanced by normal levels of circulating testosterone in the blood. By removing the source of male testosterone, the growth and spread in 90 percent of patients with prostate cancer is markedly slowed, and the cancer cells are "starved." Although not curative, the lowering of male hormone levels in the circulating blood has been proven to be an excellent palliation for patients whose cancer has spread beyond the confines of the prostate and is therefore not curable.

There are several ways to reduce circulating testosterone to near zero, but removal of the testes in an operation known as bilateral orchiectomy has been considered for many years the most effective way. This operation can be done under local anesthesia on an outpatient basis. The surgeon makes a small incision in the lower part of the scrotum, the testes are removed, and the incision is closed, leaving the scrotum intact. Sometimes, in cases where cosmetic effect is important to the patient, implantation of a testicular prosthesis is done at the same time. These prostheses are testicles made of silicone-filled gel. Although the operation is very effective, it is understandably dreaded by many men, who sometimes opt for alternative procedures. Bilateral orchiectomy does not necessarily cause impotence, and there are many men who continue to have erections after the operation, but the operation leads to a loss of sexual desire within a short time after the operation.

For patients who refuse the surgical castration, there is an alternative: "medical castration," or "medical orchiectomy." Several types of hormones are available to reduce the levels of circulating testosterone to near zero, similar to those levels of men who undergo surgical orchiectomy:

LHRH Agonists and Anti-Androgens

A recent method of reducing testosterone levels in the circulating blood is to use drugs that interfere with the hormonal signal from the brain stimulating production of testosterone by the testicles. Under normal circumstances, the brain hormone LHRH (Luteinizing Hormone Releasing Hormone) stimulates the pituitary gland to produce LH (Luteinizing Hormone), which in turn stimulates the testicles to produce male hormones. Artificial LHRH-like hormones, paradoxically, interfere with normal production of LH and therefore with the production of testosterone by the testicles. At present two drugs are widely used as once-a-month injections, Lupron and Zoladex (brand names), both of which reduce the testosterone to castrate levels. A side effect of these drugs is the production of hot flashes, which occur in 40 to 60 percent of patients, as compared to only about 10 to 15 percent of patients who are treated with orchiectomy. In addition, the use of these drugs must be kept up indefinitely, and they are very expensive. Some patients, after being injected monthly for several months or years, may decide to have an orchiectomy instead of continuing with this form of treatment. In this case, the injections will no longer be necessary.

Although removal of the testes remains the "gold standard" for palliation of prostate cancer, the monthly injection is an acceptable alternative for patients who refuse the operation.

Another class of drugs that lower circulating testosterone to virtual castrate levels are antiandrogens such as Flutamide and Cyproterone Acetate. Flutamide has been used in combination with LHRH analogues or with orchiectomy, and although it seems to prolong life by a few months, its use (in the form of tablets that must be taken three times a day) is a matter of great controversy. Ketaconazole is an antifungal drug that has been found to lower the androgen levels, but this and other similar drugs have their drawbacks and toxicities and are not used routinely.

Estrogens

The use of female hormones (estrogens) was traditionally the alternative to surgical castration, especially in the United Kingdom and the United States. They are known to lower testosterone levels and are as effective as the removal of the testes. The problem with the use of estrogens is that they tend to induce water retention and are said to increase the risk of cardiovascular problems. Since the LHRH agonists became available estrogens no longer play a primary role in the hormone manipulation of prostate cancer.

Deferred Treatment (Observation Only)

Deferred treatment, or observation only, is a method that, although commonly used and accepted in Europe, has not been popular in the United States. The patient simply comes for periodic office visits, at which time the prostate is checked by transrectal digital examination and levels of blood PSA are obtained, but no treatment is instituted unless there is a sharp increase in the PSA levels or changes occur that are indicative of progressive prostate cancer activity.

A patient with a low-grade malignancy will probably take approximately ten years to die from prostate cancer if he receives no treatment. Since the average seventy-five year-old man has statistically surpassed his life expectancy (in the United States), treatment for prostate cancer may be unnecessary, since he is likely to die of another disease first. Similarly, a patient aged seventy with significant cardiovascular disease or other serious medical problems may not benefit from prostate treatment. In contrast, a sixty-year-old, otherwise healthy man has a significantly longer life expectancy and therefore should be treated aggressively, as he has far more to lose by not being treated. The risks of observation only are that the tumor may metastasize while its benefit is the avoidance of the adverse side effects of treatment. Keeping these facts in mind, a candidate for deferred treatment is a man who:

- Has a life expectancy of less than ten additional years
- Has a low-grade, well-differentiated, and localized malignancy and stays that way.
- Can accept the risks of not receiving treatment
- Is not willing to risk potential adverse effects of aggressive therapy

Radical Prostatectomy

Radical prostatectomy is the preferred treatment for cancer of the prostate when the patient's disease is still at a stage where a long survival or cure can be anticipated. Unlike prostatectomy for BPH, where only the obstructive part of the gland is removed, in radical prostatectomy the entire prostate gland is removed, along with the seminal vesicles. After the entire prostate has been removed, the neck of the bladder is stitched directly to the urethra at a point where the prostate was detached from it. In this way, the gap created by the removal of the prostate is bridged and continuity of the lower urinary tract is reestablished. A Foley catheter is placed in the bladder and left in place for two to three weeks.

There are two common ways to approach the gland for radical prostatectomy: the perineal approach and the retropubic approach. When the perineal approach is used, an incision is made in the perineum (the area between the scrotum and the anus). The perineal approach was very popular until some fifteen years ago, when pelvic lymph node removal became a standard preliminary step for staging prior to radical prostatectomy. Since the pelvic nodes cannot be reached by a perineal incision, two incisions were required, and perineal prostatectomy was supplanted by the retropubic approach. Recently, however, since laparoscopic lymph node dissection has become available, there has been a renewed interest in this approach.

In the retropubic approach, an incision is made in the lower part of the abdomen, as in the case of retropubic prostatectomy for BPH. The main advantage of using the retropubic approach is that it allows the surgeon to remove the pelvic lymph nodes for microscopic examination, in order to determine whether there is spread of the cancer into them. Removal of the pelvic lymph nodes (pelvic lymph node dissection) is very important because, as mentioned earlier, only after these nodes are examined can the urologist be sure that the cancer has not spread and that it is still curable.

Controversy exists over whether radical prostatectomy should be performed when the lymph nodes have been found to show microscopic invasion by prostate cancer. While some urologists feel that patients should not be subjected to such major operations, with their serious potential complications, if they are not going to be cured, others believe that even if the patient is not cured, he will do much better after removal of the prostate and long-term survival is possible. In these cases, when the urologist decides to go ahead with the radical prostatectomy knowing that the lymph nodes are involved, he will also perform orchiectomy (removal of the testicles) or place the patient on some form of hormone treatment, as he would not be cured by the radical prostatectomy alone.

Radical prostatectomy is a major surgical procedure, generally taking between two and three hours, and sometimes there is significant bleed-

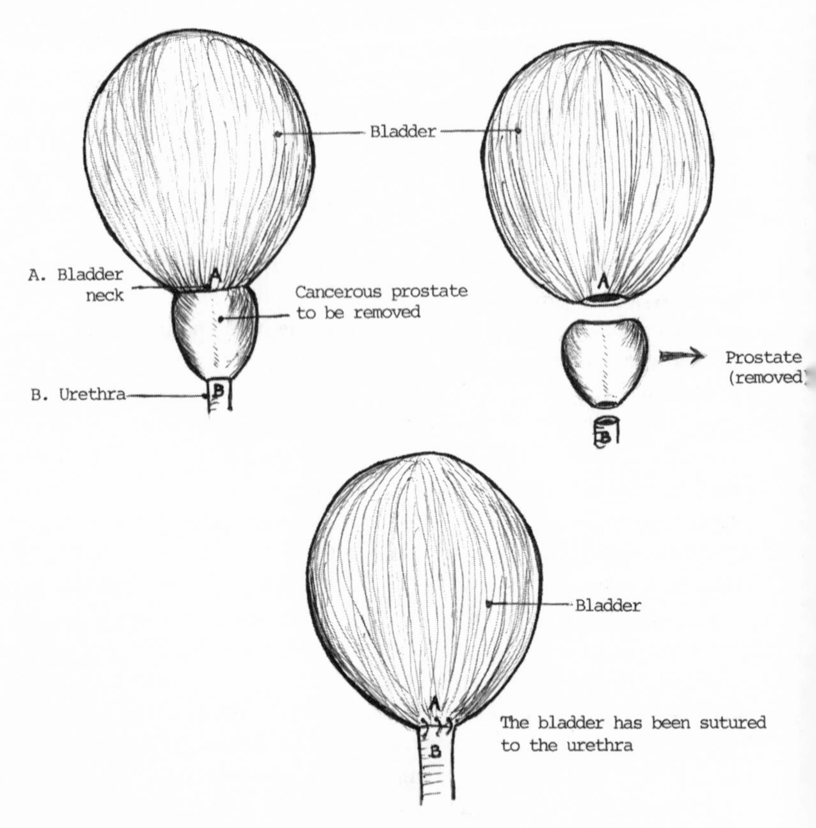

Figure 8-1. In a radical prostatectomy, the entire prostate is removed and the bladder neck is sutured to the stump of the urethra.

ing. Recovery from surgery takes longer than when prostatectomy for BPH is performed. The patient is generally hospitalized for about one week and then is sent home with a Foley catheter in place, which is removed two to three weeks after surgery, during his first postoperative office visit. The ideal candidate for radical prostatectomy is a patient who:

- Has a life expectancy of more than ten additional years
- Has a high-grade cancer
- Has disease confined to the prostate gland
- Wants the best chance of cure
- Is willing to accept the risks of surgery

Complications of Radical Prostatectomy

Radical prostatectomy is the preferred treatment to cure cancer of the prostate when it is detected early enough and is still confined to the gland. It is a major surgical procedure and, as any operation of this magnitude, carries the risk of possible complications. The most common complications are:

- Urinary incontinence
- Impotence (Erectile Dysfunction)
- Contracture of the vesical neck
- Lymphocele

Urinary Incontinence

When radical prostatectomy is performed the entire gland is removed, including the prostatic urethra. The gap created by removal of the prostate is bridged by bringing the bladder down and suturing the neck of the bladder to the remaining urethra. Since the prostatic urethra, which is several centimeters long, is removed, there is a chance of incontinence, as the prostatic urethra forms part of the continence mechanism. Although most patients have poor urinary control during the first few days after the Foley catheter is removed (two or three weeks after surgery), within the next few weeks most patients have achieved significant control. Patients are encouraged to practice the so-called Kegel exercise, which strengthens all the pelvic muscles and improves continence. The patient should exercise by tightening the muscles of the floor of the pelvis, which is exactly what he does when he wants to suddenly shut off the flow of the urinary stream. By the sixth month after surgery, the great majority of patients have normal control. If, however, incontinence persists at the end of the first year, the placement of an artificial sphincter, as described for incontinence with BPH, may be necessary.

Impotence (Erectile Dysfunction)

Until recently, the great majority of patients who underwent radical prostatectomy became impotent. But during the last decade a modification of the radical surgical procedure has been developed that spares the nerves which control erections. These nerves, which run just behind and on either side of the prostate, used to be damaged during removal of the prostate, but once urologists learned their function in controlling erections, a nerve-sparing technique was developed. When this technique is performed successfully, some patients regain the degree of potency they had prior to surgery. A few years ago, many patients who were sexually active would not accept radical prostatectomy, opting for a less effective treatment for fear of becoming impotent; but with the modified technique used now, preservation of potency is possible in a majority of patients undergoing radical prostatectomy. Potency returns more often in younger men and in patients with lower stage tumors.

Dr. Charles B. Brendler of the Johns Hopkins University, Baltimore, Maryland, studied the results of 587 consecutive men who underwent radical prostatectomy at the Johns Hopkins Hospital in 1982 and 1988, in terms of sexual function. Of those 587 patients, 503 (or 86 percent) were potent preoperatively. These patients were followed for a minimum of 18 months, and 342 (or 68 percent) were found to still be potent.

There was significant correlation between patient age and recovery of potency, compared to only 25 percent of men over 70 years of age. Potency rates also decreased with advancing clinical stage. Overall, 88 percent of patients with A_1 disease were potent compared to 59 percent of patients with B_2 disease.

Men are now more apt to choose radical prostatectomy as treatment for their prostate cancer, particularly when they know that the chance of impotence after radiation treatment could be as high as 50 percent.

Treatment of impotence that results after radical prostatectomy can involve several drugs such as papaverine, phentolamine, and prostaglandin. These drugs used alone or in combination are injected directly into the penis through a tiny needle similar to the one used by diabetics to inject themselves with insulin. The drug injections are initially done by the urologist, and if the patient is satisfied with the results, he is taught how to inject himself at home. An erection usually occurs within a few minutes after injection, and if followed by foreplay, grows firmer and may last for two hours or longer. The patient is instructed to use the injections no more than twice or three times a week. These drugs, although used extensively by most urologists, are not yet approved by the FDA for such use.

An alternative therapy is the penile prosthesis, which is implanted directly inside the spongy bodies of the penis and stiffens them to allow for penetration during intercourse (Fig. 8-2). There are many types and

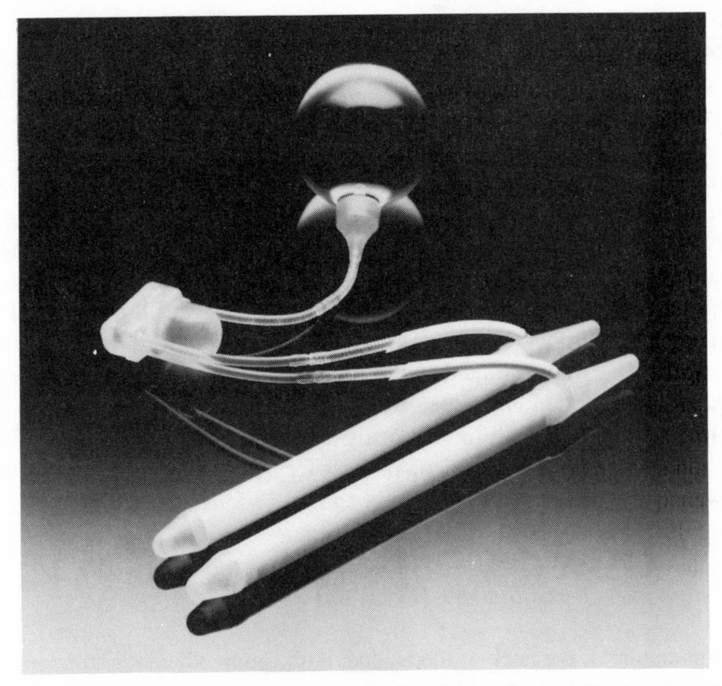

Figure 8-2. Above: An inflatable prosthesis with its three main components: inflatable cylinders, the pump, and a reservoir that contains sterile fluid. Below: The prosthesis is in place. (*Diagram courtesy American Medical Systems*)

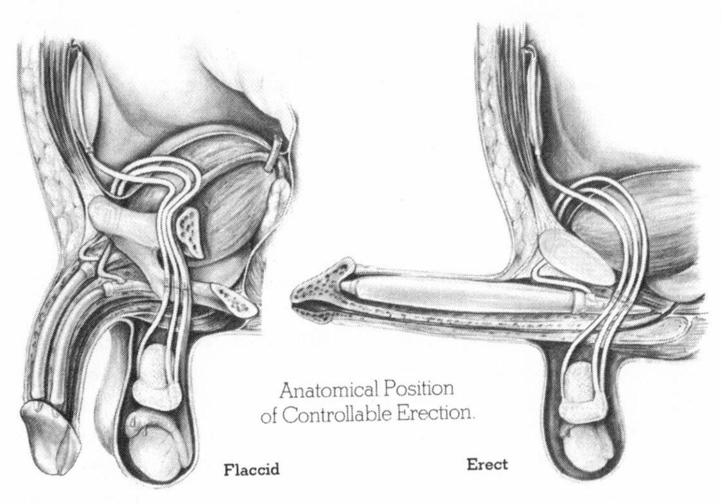

brands of prosthesis and they are either inflatable or semirigid. Each of these has advantages and disadvantages, and each should be carefully explained to the patient and his sexual partner so that they can select the prosthesis that fits their individual preferences.

Another way to treat impotence is through the use of vacuum erectile devices (Fig. 8-3). This method is safe, simple to use, and it is not permanent. Vacuum devices consist of a plastic cylinder large enough to fit over the erect penis, a hand operated vaccum pump with a special safety valve, tubing to connect the cylinder to the vacuum pump, and an elastic or seal ring can be added or removed to vary the size of the opening for proper fit. (Fig. 8-4). The device produces erection by creating a vacuum around the penis that triggers passive blood flow into the penis. Erection is maintained by the tension band or ring, which is placed around the base of the penis.

The effectiveness of vacuum devices for treating impotence has been assesed in many studies. No significant or serious complications from the use of this device have been reported.

Contracture of the Bladder Neck

Contracture of the neck of the bladder at the point where it is stitched to the urethra is a possible complication of radical prostatectomy. It generally occurs within two or three months of the operation. Typically, the patient begins to experience difficulty voiding, the caliber of his urinary stream becomes smaller, and he may have to strain to urinate. This vesical neck contracture is similar to the one that occurs after TURP for correction of obstructive BPH, and the treatment is the same. A transurethral incision through the contracted, scarred bladder neck usually works very well, and sometimes a simple dilatation with a urethral dilator may be sufficient. Once the problem is corrected it generally does not recur.

Lymphocele

Lymphocele is not a complication of radical prostatectomy, but a complication of the pelvic lymph node dissection that is generally done at the same time. A postoperative collection of lymph fluid in the pelvis, lymphocele, has been reported to occur in .5 to 10 percent of pelvic lymph node dissections for cancer of the prostate. Its prevention depends upon surgical technique and the careful ligation of lymphatic

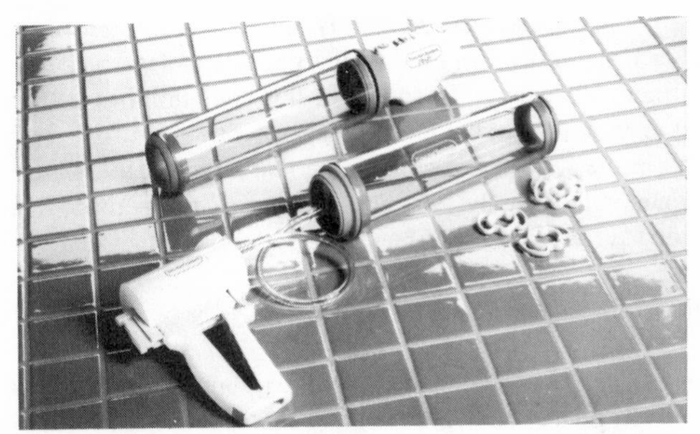

Figure 8-3. The main components of one of the many vacuum erectile devices now in use: plastic cylinders, a pump, and several constriction bands. (*Courtesy Osbon Medical Systems*)

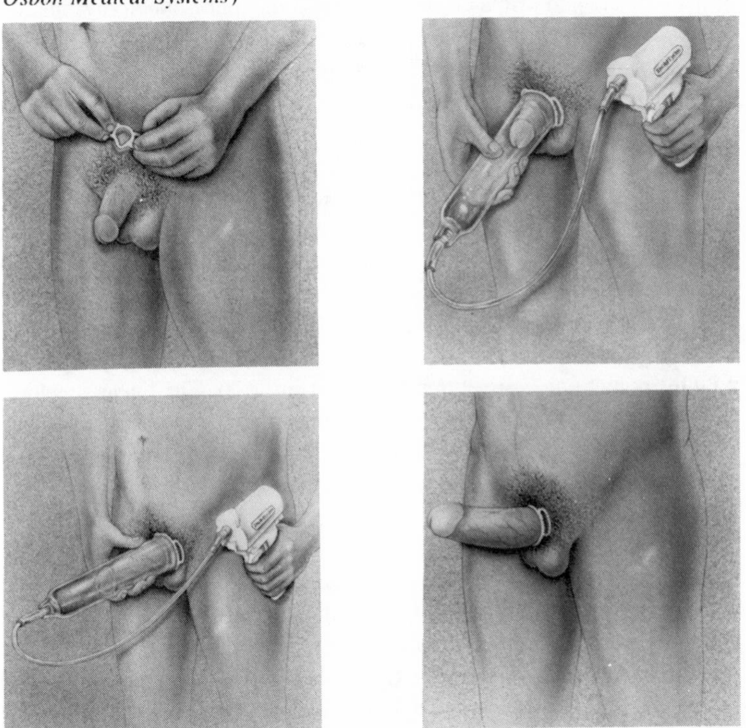

Figure 8-4. A vacuum erectile device in use. Note that the plastic cylinder has been sealed around the penis. When the pump is activated, it draws air out of the cylinder and allows blood to fill the penis. (*Courtesy Osbon Medical Systems*)

channels. Symptoms associated with lymphocele are: vague abdominal fullness or discomfort, swelling of the genitals or legs, and, in some cases, urinary frequency. Treatment of this condition has traditionally involved open drainage, but recently laparoscopy—in which a window is created in the wall of the lymphocele that allows it to drain directly into the abdominal cavity, where the lymph is reabsorbed—has produced good results.

Radiation Therapy

The basic principle of radiation therapy is to bombard the cancer with radiation at doses that damage or destroy cancer cells yet produce only a minimal amount of damage to the surrounding normal tissues. This form of therapy is used extensively in the United States to treat cancer of the prostate and offers an alternative to radical prostatectomy, mainly for those patients who are not good candidates for surgery because of their poor medical condition. There are two types of radiation therapy—external beam radiation and internal or interstitial.

External Beam Radiation

External radiation, by far the most commonly used method of radiation of prostate cancer, employs either a linear accelerator or a cobalt-60 source to pinpoint the delivery of radiation. The linear accelerator uses a much higher voltage than cobalt 60 and delivers its radiation energy below the skin level, so that skin burns, which are relatively common with the cobalt units, are extremely rare (Fig. 8-5). The linear accelerator is clearly the preferred unit for radiation, but it is twice as expensive as the cobalt unit, and this difference in price is the reason that the cobalt units arc still used in some institutions.

Radiation is generally given in daily sessions five times a week over a period of six to seven weeks. The number of treatments and the dose of radiation depend upon the size of the prostate, the extent of the disease, and the physical condition of the patient. However, the dosage is generally between 6,500 and 7,000 rads (units of measurement of the amount of radiation delivered). Radiation is given over a period of time because it must be strong enough to kill the cancer and still allow the normal radiated tissue to heal. Although some normal cells surrounding the cancer will suffer radiation damage, they recover between treatments.

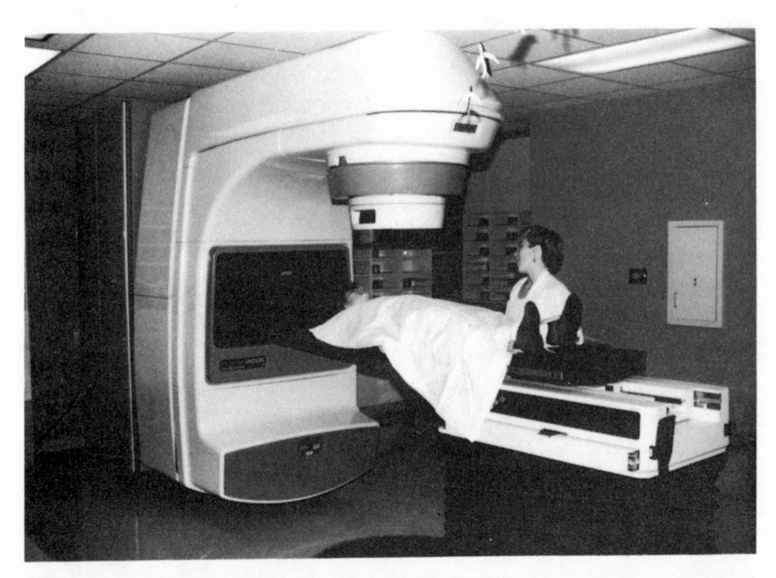

Figure 8-5. A modern linear accelerator used in the treatment with external radiation. (*Courtesy Northern Virginia Cancer Center*)

Internal (Interstitial) Radiation

In this method, radioactive pellets or seeds are inserted into the prostate through long needles. An incision is made in the lower part of the abdomen in the same manner as in a radical prostatectomy, and pelvic lymph nodes are removed for microscopic examination for presence of tumor cells. Several needles are then placed in the prostate, through which the pellets or seeds are implanted. Although this method was very popular about ten years ago, it is only rarely done today, mainly because of improvement in the technique of radical prostatectomy and because placement of internal radiation seeds subjected the patient to an increased risk of complications—those of open surgery and anesthesia plus risk of complications from radiation.

More recently, transrectal ultrasound-guided placement of radioactive seeds into the prostate gland has received some attention, since it eliminates the need for an operation and is less time-consuming for the patient, as well as the medical staff. The disadvantage of this modality is that tumors with ill-defined margins may not be adequately irradiated and lymph node involvement cannot be determined. Far more research, experience, and follow-up are needed before this method gains wide acceptance, but preliminary reports are encouraging. An ideal candidate for radiation would be a man who:

- Has a life expectancy of ten years or more
- Has a high-grade cancer
- Wants to avoid surgery
- Can accept the uncertainty about the possible persistence of cancer
- Wants to receive some kind of treatment
- Is willing to accept the risks of radiation

Radiation for Advanced Cancer

There is significant controversy over the role of radiation therapy in Stage D prostate cancer patients. Once prostate cancer is in the lymph nodes it cannot be cured, but there are some radiotherapists who feel that radiation produces better local control of the disease. The overall survival of patients with Stage D_1 disease after radiation therapy is poor—not different, in fact, from that found when no treatment at all is given. Radiation is frequently used with good results in the treatment of painful bone metastasis, particularly in the spine. This form of therapy, although not curative, is an excellent means of pain control in some cases.

Side Effects From Radiation

One of the most common side effects of radiation therapy is diarrhea. It generally responds well to medications, but sometimes is very persistent and may have periodic flare-ups for years after the treatment. Occasionally, a serious rectal injury such as perforation or obstruction may occur. Fortunately, this is rare, occurring in less than 1 percent of cases. Other side effects may be loss of appetite, nausea, vomiting, or symptoms of cystitis, such as frequency, urgency, and painful urination. Although most of these symptoms disappear, some patients develop radiation cystitis—which may not become symptomatic for several years, and by which time recurrent bleeding on urination and, occasionally, permanent damage to the bladder may have occurred. If complications occur, they are sometimes permanent.

Impotence is a significant complication from radiation of the prostate and the American Cancer Society estimates that it occurs in 30 to 50 percent of patients within two years of treatment. The cause of this distressing complication is not clear, but it is probably due to the effect of the radiation on the blood vessels supplying the spongy part of the penis. Urinary incontinence is not common, but it occurs, particularly in patients who have had previous prostate operations, such as TURP. In general, radiation is well tolerated and the common belief that people get very ill from it is not true, although most patients do complain of fatigue. Nonetheless, the majority of them are able to work and enjoy leisure activities while undergoing radiation therapy.

It is rare for a patient to have to stop treatment because of side effects. Superficial skin burns are rare with the linear accelerator, and generally respond well to local treatment. Some pubic hair loss may occur, and the skin may turn a shade darker. However, these changes are to be expected and patients should not be concerned about them. Recommendations for minimizing side effects are to get plenty of rest and eat a well-balanced diet (avoiding dieting and weight-loss programs while undergoing treatment).

CHAPTER 9

Prostatitis: Infections and Inflammations of the Prostate

Prostatitis is a general term used to cover various types of inflammation of the prostate. It is generally caused by invasion of the prostate by bacteria. In its various forms, prostatitis is certainly very common, particularly between the ages of thirty and fifty, although it can occur in adult males of any age. Prostatitis generally causes a great deal of anxiety, worry, and, frequently, concern over the possibility of having a venereal disease. There are several types of prostatitis:

- Acute bacterial prostatitis
- Chronic bacterial prostatitis
- Nonbacterial prostatitis
- Stress prostatitis (prostatodynia, prostatosis)

Acute Bacterial Prostatitis

Acute bacterial prostatitis results from a rather sudden invasion of bacteria into the prostate gland. The route by which bacteria reach the prostate is largely unknown, but possibilities include the ascension of infection through the urethra, by means of the bloodstream, from a focus of infection in a distant part of the body such as skin, tonsils, or teeth, or bacteria introduced from the rectum, which is located next to the prostate. Instrumentation of the urethra or the bladder such as cystoscopy, dilatation of the urethra, or just the passing of a catheter into the bladder are known causes of prostatitis, and for this reason physicians frequently use antibiotics after such instrumentations. The bacteria that cause acute prostatitis are mainly those that normally colonize the large bowel and urinary tract (coliform bacteria), but occasionally other types of bacteria may be involved.

Acute bacterial prostatitis is the most dramatic form of prostatitis, but it is also the form that responds best to treatment. Patients with acute prostatitis feel quite sick and generally run a high fever, and usually seek medical attention rapidly, especially when the act of voiding becomes difficult or impossible. Following recovery, the condition rarely recurs.

Symptoms

Symptoms of acute bacterial prostatitis include:

- Fever and chills
- Urinary frequency and urgency
- Painful urination
- Blood in the urine
- Generalized malaise, flu-like symptoms
- Pain in the area between the scrotum and the anus
- Difficulty voiding and sometimes even acute retention

All of these are common symptoms; as a result of them, patients frequently feel as though they are sitting on something hard, "like a golf ball," and may experience severe pain.

Diagnosis

The diagnosis is generally made using clinical history, laboratory findings, and physical examination. The prostate is generally very tender to palpation and very painful. The findings are frequently striking and the diagnosis simple to make. A midstream urine specimen will invariably show over 100,000 bacterial colonies per cubic millimeter of urine.

Treatment

Acute bacterial prostatitis frequently responds dramatically to antibiotic treatment. The intense and diffuse swelling of the prostate is thought by some to facilitate the penetration of antibiotics into it. In addition to antibiotics, which frequently need to be given intravenously in a hospital setting, adequate hydration is necessary, analgesics are administered as needed for pain, bed rest is strongly recommended, and, in some cases, stool softeners are used. In severe cases, when there is marked swelling of the prostate, the patient may become unable to urinate as in the case of obstructive BPH, and may require the passage of a small catheter into the bladder to relieve the temporary obstruction.

Chronic Bacterial Prostatitis

The term chronic means long-lasting. Unlike acute bacterial prostatitis, chronic bacterial prostatitis does not generally cause acute or dramatic onset of severe symptoms. These develop gradually over a period of time, during which patients generally do not feel very ill and are able to function in their normal activities. Many cases of chronic prostatitis follow an episode of acute prostatitis, but it more commonly develops for no apparent reason.

Symptoms

Symptoms, when present, are generally milder than in acute prostatitis, and usually are:

- Frequent, and sometimes difficult, urination
- Urgent need to urinate
- Pain in the pelvis, genital, lower back, or lower abdomen
- Painful ejaculation; sometimes, blood in the semen
- Occasionally, low-grade fever

These symptoms, although not severe, can be very incapacitating. Many patients with chronic prostatitis, however, may have no symptoms at all.

Diagnosis

Diagnosing chronic bacterial prostatitis is not as easy as diagnosing acute bacterial prostatitis. As in the case of acute prostatitis, the diagnosis is made on the basis of a careful clinical history, a physical examination, and laboratory tests on the urine. A culture of urine is necessary to diagnose chronic prostatitis. To collect a urine sample, the so-called 3-glass technique is used. The patient is asked to begin urinating into a glass marked 1; then, without interrupting his stream, he is asked to void an equal amount into a glass marked 2; then, again without interrupting his stream, he can void into the toilet, but he is asked to retain some urine in his bladder. The physician asks the patient to bend over and massages his prostate through the rectum. When infection is present, this is painful; the massage drains the prostate, and the secretions generally pool in the prostatic urethra. The patient is then asked to void into a glass marked 3.

The contents of the three glasses are then cultured. Glass 2 will be sterile, unless a bladder infection is present. A definitive diagnosis of chronic bacterial prostatitis can be made if there is at least a tenfold increase in the bacterial colony count obtained from the urine in glass 3 as compared to 1. A high bacterial count in glass 1 suggests a urethral infection, rather than chronic prostatitis. When the bacteria colony count in glass 3 is no higher than in 1, nonspecific urethritis is the most likely diagnosis.

TREATMENT.

Chronic bacterial prostatitis is difficult to cure. As we have seen in Chapter 1, the prostate is a rather complex organ, composed of many tiny sacs that are lined with cells that secrete fluid, which drain into innumerable small ducts and finally into the urethra through several tiny exits. Once bacteria begin to grow in this dense network of glands, sacs, and tubules they are hard to eradicate, since the antibiotics carried by way of the bloodstream may not be able to penetrate into every little sac and cavity of the prostate. Another factor that makes cure of chronic prostatitis difficult is the presence of tiny calculi (stones) that are frequently formed in the prostate. Although these calculi occur in almost every adult prostate and generally cause no symptoms or harm, in certain men with chronic bacterial prostatitis, the calculi may become infected and are the source of bacterial persistance. Antibiotics cannot penetrate these stones, and it is only a matter of time before the infection flares up again once the antibiotics have been discontinued.

The primary approach in the treatment of chronic bacterial prostatitis is to attempt to cure the infection with antibiotics, which may be required for as long as three months. Newly available drugs have shown great promise in the eradication of chronic bacterial prostatitis. In an effort to obtain sufficient concentration of the antibiotic within the prostate, direct intraprostatic injection of antibiotic agents has been used by one group of investigators, but the long-term results have not been encouraging.

Sometimes, if long-term use of antibiotics fails to cure the disease, transurethral resection of the prostate, as done for BPH, may be helpful, particularly when stones are present in the prostate. In some cases, however, even a generous TURP fails to cure the infection; only about a third of patients are cured by this procedure. Hot sitz baths frequently provide relief from the pain. Periodic prostatic massages have been used for years to drain secretions from the prostate, but it is the author's view that this is a poor substitute for ejaculation, which does a far better job of emptying the prostate.

This is frequently a very frustrating condition, and the patient needs to understand what is happening. He needs to know that there is no magic cure and that treatment may take quite some time. The doctor needs to be very sympathetic and to give him all possible support.

Nonbacterial Prostatitis

Unlike the two previous types of prostatitis, with this type there is no bacteria that can be cultured or identified as the cause of the inflammation. Urine cultures obtained after a prostate massage are typically negative, although inflammatory cells and other signs of inflammation may be present.

A variety of microorganisms has been blamed as the cause of this condition, such as viruses, viruslike organisms, and chlamydiae, but attempts at demonstrating this causal relationship have not been conclusive. A common belief among urologists is that the condition may result from engorgement of the fluid-producing small glands within the prostate. The prostate gland is normally emptied during ejaculation by spasmodic contraction of the muscles around it. If a man is used to having sexual intercourse on a regular basis, say once or more every week, and this regularity is then interrupted, the prostate gland will begin to retain fluids, causing the prostate to become engorged, congested, and inflamed.

There has been some suggestion that chronic nonbacterial, or congestive prostatitis may be brought about or made worse by jogging or doing heavy lifting with a full bladder, as this would force urine to reflux, or flow back, through the small openings of the prostatic urethra into the prostate, and cause chemical inflammation.

Chronic vibration has been blamed as the cause of some cases of nonbacterial prostatitis. Men whose occupations expose them to chronic vibrations, such as bus or taxi drivers, appear to be prone to develop this problem. These patients seem to do better when they try to empty their prostates by ejaculating more often.

Coitus interruptus has also been blamed as a contributing factor in developing nonbacterial prostatitis. Coitus interruptus is the most widely used form of contraception, since it requires no advanced planning or expense. But the fact is that this form of contraception is very unreliable, because prior to ejaculation men frequently dribble small amounts of fluid containing enough sperm to impregnate a fertile woman. Coitus interruptus may also cause engorgement of the prostate.

Symptoms.

The symptoms of nonbacterial prostatitis are very similar to those of chronic prostatitis, and in many ways these two conditions are similar. The only difference is that in nonbacterial prostatitis the inflammation has never been proven to be caused by any bacteria.

Diagnosis

Since the symptoms of chronic prostatitus are similar to those of nonbacterial prostatitus, obtaining a complete clinical history is very important. The possibility of chronic prostatitus has to be ruled out by obtaining adequate urine cultures. Once this is done, one can consider the possibility of non-bacterial prostatitus. It is important to establish the proper diagnosis because the treatment would be different.

Treatment.

Predictably, effective treatment for nonbacterial prostatitis is not available, since the cause is not known. Antimicrobial therapy for two weeks with tetracycline or doxycycline, which are effective against C. trachomatis and U. urealyticum, is a reasonable initial approach and has been effective in some cases. Several reports have documented the value of these and other similar antibiotic treatments in some men with nonbacterial prostatitis.

Long-term use of antimicrobials is discouraged, as evidence for an infectious cause of nonbacterial prostatitis is limited at best, and the toxicity of these drugs when used for a long time is therefore not justifiable. Hot sitz baths, anti-inflammatory drugs, or mild tranquilizers may occasionally prove beneficial.

Stress Prostatitis

Stress prostatitis (also called prostatodynia and prostatosis) is a very common condition that has baffled urologists for years and is one of the greatest enigmas in medicine. Although not a serious condition, it has brought incredible aggravation, misery, anxiety, and frustration to millions of unfortunate men. The term "stress prostatitis" was first used by Dr. Harry C. Miller, chairman of the Department of Urology at George Washington University in Washington, D.C., after he studied 218 men with symptoms of this condition and reported his findings in the December 1988 issue of *Urology* (vol. 32, no. 6), Dr. Miller concluded that the symptoms were due to changes in the prostate caused by stress. It is known that when the automatic nervous system is stimulated by stress it responds with a variety of symptoms caused by changes that take place in such target organs as the stomach, colon, bronchial tree (divisions of subdivisions of bronchi), and blood vessels. The prostate has the same autonomic nerve fibers as many of these organs. Stimulation of the prostate by these fibers results in prostatic fluid secretion and contraction of the muscular fibers within the prostate, which Dr. Miller believes are responsible for the symptoms. He identified the prostate as a target organ for stress, and this recognition has opened an entirely new dimension in our understanding of this condition.

Symptoms

The symptoms are in many ways similar to those of chronic bacterial prostatitis, but there is no infection present and examination of the urine shows no abnormalities. Symptoms are generally:

- Discomfort, aching, or pain in the genitalia, lower abdomen, pelvis, or prostate, generally at the end of voiding

- Low back pain
- Discomfort on ejaculation
- Urinary frequency, and a great urge to urinate
- Thin, watery early-morning urethral discharge
- Feelings of anxiety, worry, guilt, and anger

These symptoms generally occur intermittently for months or years. Most patients become "physician shoppers," going from doctor to doctor in the hope that one of them may end their misery. They are frustrated and anxious, and their anxiety is increased after a battery of laboratory tests and other diagnostic procedures produce only negative results. Some begin to feel that they may have a serious condition such as cancer of the prostate or, more recently, AIDS. If they have had an extramarital affair, feelings of guilt develop, increasing their anxiety level and the intensity of their symptoms, and sometimes causing poor erections. Dr. Miller's patients who were identified as having stress prostatitis were given no other treatment besides reassurance, explanation of their condition, and stress management instructions. They were sent on their way with no prescription, no prostatic massages, and no plans for X rays or other testing. Of the 218 patients studied in 1988 and followed, 86 percent indicated that they were "better," "much better," or "cured" when seen two years later. In recent personal communication, Dr. Miller stated that the number of his patients in the study is now near 400 and that 89 percent of them show significant improvement or are cured, and that a follow-up will soon be reported.

Although not every urologist agrees with this form of therapy, during the past two years the author has had the opportunity to treat many patients with this condition, and the great majority of them have reported excellent results. Patients feel a great deal of relief when they are reassured that they do not suffer from a serious condition, that their problem is not due to a contagious disease, and that there is no need to do elaborate diagnostic testing. Most of them admit that they'd suspected stress had played a significant role in their symptoms, and are very willing to follow directions. It is entirely likely that stress prostatitis is responsible for some cases of nonbacterial prostatitis.

Glossary

Acid Phosphatase An enzyme made in the prostate gland.

Acute Reaching a crisis rapidly; having a short and severe course; sudden.

Adenoma A benign tumor in which the cells form glandular structures.

Ampulla A dilatation in a canal or duct.

Androgens Masculine hormones that encourage the development of male sexual characteristics.

Anesthesia A loss of feeling or sensation. In general anesthesia, there is loss of consciousness produced by an anesthetic agent that causes absence of pain sensation over the entire body. In the case of local anesthesia, the loss of pain sensation is localized in one part of the body. In epidural and spinal anesthesia the loss of sensation occurs from the waist down.

Antihistamine Any of a group of drugs used to relieve symptoms of allergies and colds. They work by neutralizing the effect of histamine, an active substance in allergic reactions.

Anus The opening found at the end of the digestive tract.

Artificial urinary sphincter A prosthesis designed to restore continence in an incontinent person by compressing the urethra.

Aspiration The removal of fluids, gases, or cells by the application of suction. Aspiration needle biopsy is done by using suction through a syringe.

Bacteria Unicellular microorganisms that may cause infection.

Bacterial prostatitus Infection of the prostate gland caused by bacteria.

Bacteriuria The presence of bacteria in the urine.

Benign Nonmalignant.

Benign prostate hypertrophy (BPH) The nonmalignant but abnormal multiplication of prostate cells in prostate tissue.

Bilateral Having two sides.

Biopsy A procedure whereby tissue is removed for microscopic examination to establish a precise diagnosis.

Bladder An elastic sac that serves to store urine. The term is used to designate the urinary bladder.

Bladder catheterization Passage of a catheter into the urinary bladder.

Bladder neck contracture An abnormal narrowing and scarring of the bladder neck that interferes with passage of urine. Can be a complication of prostate surgery.

Bladder outlet The first portion of the channel through which urine flows from the bladder.

Bladder outlet obstruction Obstruction of the bladder outlet, commonly caused by prostate enlargement.

Bladder spasm A sudden and involuntary contraction of the bladder wall, causing pain and an urge to urinate.

Bone scan A picture of the bones obtained after the patient has been injected with a radioactive substance, which concentrates in the bones. It is particularly used to diagnose prostate cancer that has metastasized to bones.

BPH See Benign prostate hypertrophy.

Cancer Disorderly and uncontrolled growth of abnormal cells, the natural course of which is fatal. Also called malignant tumor or malignancy.

Capsule The structure in which something is enclosed.

Castration In men, the removal of the testicles by surgery. Chemical castration is the suppression of male hormones by chemical means.

Catheter A tubular, flexible instrument designed to be passed through the urethra into the bladder in order to drain urine.

CAT scan Also known as a CT scan, or computerized axial tomography, a diagnostic technique that utilizes computers and X rays to obtain a highly detailed image of the section of the body being studied.

Cervix Opening of the uterus.

Chemotherapy Treatment of cancer with drugs that can interfere with the growth of cancer cells.

Chlamydia A family of small bacterial organisms that frequently cause infections in the urethra.

Chronic Of long duration. Chronic bacterial prostatitis is an infection of the prostate that persists over a long period of time.

Coitus Sexual intercourse.

Coitus interruptus Conscious withdrawal of the penis prior to ejaculation.

Coitus prolongus Conscious postponement of ejaculation and orgasm.

Congestion Swelling due to the presence of increased blood supply.

Congestive prostatitis Also known as prostatodynia and prostatosis, a noninfectious form of prostatitis.

Contracture (bladder neck) See bladder neck contracture.

Contrast medium A dye injected into a vein to highlight internal structures through X rays.

Creatinine A normal waste product filtered by the kidneys, the measurement of which in the blood is an excellent indication of kidney function.

Cystoscope An instrument used for the internal examination of the bladder and urethra.

Cystoscopy Internal visual examination of the bladder and urethra, done with a cystoscope.

Decompensated bladder A bladder that does not empty after voiding and loses its ability to contract.

Digital rectal examination DRE (Prostate) An examination of the prostate by inserting a gloved, well-lubricated finger into the rectum.

Diverticulum A pouch or sac protruding out from a hollow organ such as the bladder.

Dribbling An involuntary loss of urine that occurs in drops, generally at the conclusion of voiding.

-ectomy A suffix meaning "surgical removal," as in prostatectomy.

Ejaculate The semen expelled in ejaculation.

Ejaculatory duct The tubular structure through which the semen reaches the prostatic urethra.

Enucleation The removal or shelling out of a tumor from the structure that contains it, like a nut from its shell.

Enzymes Proteins produced by living cells that help to produce chemical reactions.

Epididymis A cordlike structure along the posterior border of the testicle that provides storage and maturation of sperm.

Epididymitis Inflammation of the epididymis.

Erection The enlargement and stiffening of the penis when it becomes filled with blood.

Estrogen A general name for the female sex hormone made in the ovaries.

Estrogen therapy The use of estrogens in the treatment of prostate cancer.

Excretory urogram See IVP.

External Urethral Sphincter Circular muscular structure which wraps around the urethra, located just below the prostate, and responsible for urinary control.

External radiation Radiation emitted by a radiation machine directed toward the diseased part of the body.

False negative The erroneous result of a test when it is reported as negative, but is truly positive.

False positive The erroneous result of a test when it is reported as positive, but is truly negative.

Fertile Capable of conceiving and bearing children.

Flow rate (urine) The measurement of the force and caliber of the urinary stream. If it is abnormal, it may be indicative of obstruction.

Foley catheter A catheter that is placed in the bladder for continuous drainage and is kept in place by means of a balloon inflated within the bladder.

Fossa A hollowed-out place.

Frequency (urinary) The desire to urinate very often.

Genitals The male and female reproductive organs, internal and external.

Gland An aggregation of cells that secrete and excrete a substance.

Grading (cancer) The determination of the degree of malignancy, based on microscopic evidence.

Hematuria The presence of blood in the urine.

Hesitancy Delayed initiation of the urinary stream.

Hormonal therapy The treatment of cancer with hormones, or hormone manipulation.

Hormone A chemical substance produced by an endocrine gland and carried by the bloodstream.

Hyperplasia The nonmalignant but abnormal multiplication of cells. Also known as Hypertrophy.

Hyperplastic (prostatic tissue) See Benign prostate hypertrophy.

Hypertrophy See Hyperplasia

Hypoechoic (less echogenic) Prostate cancer frequently appears as a hypoechoic area prostate sonogram.
Impotence Inability to initiate or maintain an erection.
Incontinence Inability to control the discharge of urine.
Induration Firmness. Areas of prostate induration may be due to cancer.
Indwelling catheterization Catheterization of the bladder with a catheter that stays in the bladder for continuous drainage.
Infection Invasion of a body part by microorganisms, resulting in injury to tissues.
Inflammation A condition resulting from injury, infection, or irritation. This condition is characterized by redness, heat, swelling, and pain.
Intermittent catheterization Catheterization on a systematic-interval schedule.
Internal Sphincter Circular, muscular fibers around the vesical neck.
IVP (Intravenous pyelogram) A series of X-ray pictures taken after a contrast material has been injected into the patient's bloodstream. This contrast material is eliminated through the kidneys and outlines the urinary tract.
Lesion A wound, an injury, or a mass, which may be solid or cystic, benign or malignant.
Local anesthesia See Anesthesia.
Lymph nodes Small bean-shaped masses of tissue that act as filters, filtering toxins, bacteria, and tumor cells. They are also a common site for cancer spread.
Male hormones Substances produced by the testes and other glands that are responsible for the male sexual characteristics. Testosterone is the main male hormone.
Male reproductive system The system of the body concerned with the production, maturation, and transport of sperm.
Malignant Cancerous. Having the properties of invasion and metastasis as applied to tumors.
Metastatic cancer Cancer that has spread from the original organ to other parts of the body.
Metastases The spread or colonization of an original cancerous tumor to other parts of the body.
MRI (Magnetic resonance imaging) A test similar to CT scanning but in which the patient is not exposed to any radiation and there is no known hazard. It produces imaging of a particular body section.
Neck of the bladder. Also known as vesical neck, is the opening of the bladder into the prostatic urethra.
Needle biopsy Biopsy obtained through a special needle.
Nocturia Being awakened at night by a desire to urinate.
Nodule A small lump, generally malignant.
Nonbacterial prostatitis Inflection of the prostate gland in the absence of any demonstrable bacterial microorganism.
Occult prostatic carcinoma Cancer of the prostate that is neither suspected nor diagnosed but is discovered after prostate surgery for BPH. It is also called Stage A prostate cancer.

Orchiectomy The surgical removal of the testes.
Orgasm The climax of the sexual act, usually accompanied by muscular contractions and ejaculation.
Overflow incontinence The condition in which the bladder remains virtually full after voiding, and urine "spills over."
Peak urinary flow rate The maximum rate of urinary flow that the patient is able to generate.
Penile prosthesis A synthetic material that is inserted into the spongy bodies of the penis so as to make the penis rigid enough for vaginal penetration.
Perineal Pertaining to the perineum, the area of the body between the scrotum and the anus.
Potency The ability of a man to achieve and maintain an erection sufficient for penetration.
Prognosis The forecast of the probable outcome of a disease.
Prostaglandins A group of fluids produced by the prostate.
Prostate Also referred to as the prostate gland, a gland in the male that surrounds the neck of the bladder and the urethra. It secretes a fluid that forms part of the semen.
Prostate secretions The fluid that is produced in the prostate gland.
Prostatectomy Surgical removal of part of the prostate. The three most common types performed are transurethral, suprapubic, and retropubic. Radical prostatectomy is the removal of the entire prostate along with the seminal vesicles.
Prostatic adenoma See Adenoma.
Prostatic biopsy See Biopsy.
Prostatic fossa See Fossa.
Prostatic massage Transrectal massage of the prostate performed with the index finger, for the purpose of obtaining secretions from the prostate gland.
Prostatic urethra The portion of the urethra that goes through the prostate gland. It begins at the bladder neck and ends at the external urethral sphincter.
Prostatism Symptoms caused by obstructive BPH.
Prostatitis, acute, bacterial An acute inflammation of the prostate caused by bacterial infection.
Prostatitis, chronic, bacterial A long-standing inflammation of the prostate gland caused by bacterial infection.
Prostatitis, nonbacterial An inflammation of the prostate gland that is not due to bacterial infection.
Prostatodynia Also known as prostatosis; see Stress prostatitis.
Prosthesis, penile See Penile prosthesis.
Pubic bone Bone located just above the penis that forms part of the pelvis.
Radiation The process of emitting radiant energy in the form of X, light, ultraviolet, or any other electromagnetic rays from one source or center.
Radical prostatectomy See Prostatectomy.
Radiotherapy The use of radiation in the treatment of disease.
Resection (transurethral) The removal of obstructive BPH prostate tissue, done through the urethra.

Resectoscope The instrument that is used for a transurethral resection.

Residual urine Urine left behind in the bladder after voiding. Under normal circumstances there should be no residual urine.

Retention (urinary) The inability to void when the bladder is full. This is frequently due to obstructive BPH.

Retrograde ejaculation The flow of semen backward into the bladder instead of forward through the penis. This phenomenon is a frequent result of prostate surgery.

Retropubic The area behind and below the pubic bone.

Retropubic prostatectomy Surgical removal of the prostate adenoma. In this procedure the prostate is approached through the lower part of the abdomen and from behind the pubic bone.

Scan Computerized picture of an organ or body part, such as bones, liver, or brain.

Scrotum The external sac of skin that contains the testicles.

Secretions (prostatic) The fluid that is produced by the many smaller glands within the prostate.

Semen A thick, whiteish fluid that contains spermatozoa. It is a mixture of secretions from the prostate, seminal vesicles, and other minor glands.

Seminal vesicles Two sacs or pouches that are located just behind the bladder. The secretion of the seminal vesicles forms part of the semen.

Sexual dysfunction A less-than-normal sexual functioning, such as inability to obtain or maintain an erection, or inability to ejaculate.

Silent prostatism A condition in which prostatic obstruction exists without symptoms, and which can lead to serious kidney damage if not treated.

Sitz bath A regular or therapeutic hot bath in which the person sits down. This can have a palliative effect on perineal pain or discomfort.

Sonogram A computer picture that uses ultrasound (high-frequency sound waves) to examine different organs of the body.

Spasm (bladder) A sudden, violent, and involuntary contraction of the bladder wall that is generally painful and that produces an urgent desire to urinate.

Spermatozoa The mature male germ cell, produced by the testicles and capable of fertilizing the ovum (female sex cell).

Sphincter (urinary) The ringlike muscle that a man voluntarily contracts when he wants to shut off his urinary stream.

Spongy bodies A term used for the two corpora cavernosa, which are the structures within the penis that become engorged with blood during erection.

Staging (prostate cancer) The process by which one can determine whether or not a prostatic cancer is still confined within the prostate gland or has spread outside of it.

Sterile Unable to produce offspring.

Stone (bladder) Substance formed by crystallization of urine that remains in the bladder.

Stress prostatitis A condition also known by other names, such as prostatodynia, prostatosis, and congestive prostatitis. The symptoms are very similar to those caused by bacterial prostatitis, but in this condition no infective bacteria have been identified, and it is thought to be caused by stress.

Stricture (urethral) A scarring or narrowing within the urethra that causes symptoms of voiding difficulty similar to those of obstructive BPH. The stricture can be caused by an injury to the urethra.

Suprapubic Referring to the area of the abdomen above the pubic bone.

Suprapubic prostatectomy The removal of the prostate adenoma through an incision made on the skin below the navel and slightly above the pubic in the lower abdomen. In this operation the prostate is removed through an incision in the bladder.

Surgical capsule (prostate) Not a capsule at all but simply the normal prostate compressed into a thin layer of tissue between the prostatic hyperplasia and the true prostate capsule.

Suture Surgical stitches bringing together two surfaces.

Testicles Also known as testes, the two male reproductive glands that produce sperm and male hormones. They are enclosed in the scrotum.

Testosterone A hormone that encourages the development of male sex characteristics.

Therapy Remedial treatment of a disease. Estrogen or hormonal therapy indicates treatment of prostate cancer by reducing the male hormone to castrate levels.

Tissue A collection of similar specialized cells united in the performance of a particular function.

Tomography A diagnostic technique using computers and X rays to obtain a highly detailed image of a section of the body.

Trabeculation (of the bladder wall) The irregular buildup of bladder muscle that gives the inside of the bladder the appearance of Swiss cheese. This is strong evidence of bladder outlet obstruction, usually due to BPH.

Transurethral The route through the urethra. The term generally applies to something being passed into or through the urethra, such as a catheter, a cystoscope, or a resectoscope.

Transurethral prostatectomy The transrethral resection of the part of the prostate which is causing obstruction.

Transurethral resection Surgical removal of tissue, accomplished by passing an instrument through the urethra.

True capsule The fibrous layer of tissue that surrounds the prostate tissue.

Tumor Enlargement due to abnormal overgrowth of tissue. Tumors can be either benign or malignant.

Ultrasound See sonogram.

Uremic poisoning (uremia) The failure of the kidneys to eliminate excessive by-products of protein metabolism in the blood, which causes a toxic condition to develop.

Ureter The long, narrow tube through which urine passes from the kidneys into the bladder.

Urethra The muscular tube or canal through which urine passes from the bladder to the exterior of the body. In men, seminal fluid and urine pass through the urethra.

Urethral meatus Opening at the end of the urethra.

Urethral stricture See stricture.

Urethritis (nonspecific) An infection of the prostatic urethra that can be caused by any microorganism, except the gonococcus, which causes gonorrhea. The term is used to indicate that the inflammation of the urethra is not due to gonorrhea.

Urgency Acute desire to urinate, sometimes accompanied by a sensation of impending leakage.

Urine Fluid that is excreted by the kidneys, stored in the bladder, and expelled through the urethra.

Urine analysis The physical, chemical, and microscopic analysis and examination of the urine.

Urine culture The incubation of urine at a specific temperature and in a specific medium so as to permit the growth and identification of microorganisms. This is the means by which an infection in the urinary tract is diagnosed.

Urologist A physician who specializes in the medical and surgical treatment of diseases of the urinary tract in males and females and the reproductive tract in males. A urologist has had at least five years of hospital training after graduation from medical school.

Vas deferens The muscular, tubular structure that propels and transports spermatozoa from the epididymis into the prostatic urethra.

Weak urinary stream A voided stream that has less than normal expulsive force to it.

X rays Electromagnetic vibrations of short wavelengths that can penetrate most substances of the body, thus revealing the presence of fractured bones or foreign bodies.

Index

ABOUT THE AUTHOR

Dr. Hernando Salcedo served in the U.S. Navy as a medical officer and was associate professor of urology at George Washington University in Washington, D.C. He was president of the medical staff at Circle Terrace Hospital in Alexandria, Virginia and is now in private practice in Virginia.